SUPERCHARGED
JUICE & SMOOTHIE RECIPES

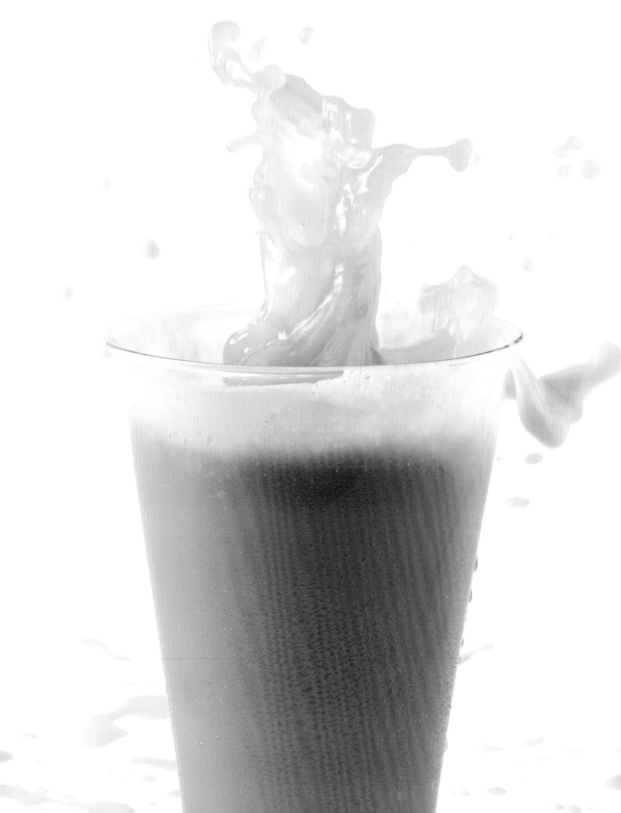

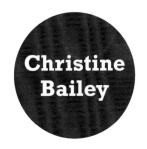

Christine Bailey

SUPERCHARGED
JUICE & SMOOTHIE RECIPES

Your Ultra-Healthy Plan for Weight Loss, Detox, Beauty & More
Using Super-Supplements

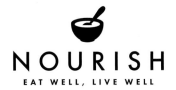

NOURISH
EAT WELL, LIVE WELL

To my wonderful husband Chris and my smoothie-loving boys Nathan, Isaac and Simeon for taste-testing every recipe many times and for providing me with love and support throughout writing this book.

Supercharged Juice & Smoothie Recipes
Christine Bailey

First published in the United Kingdom and Ireland
in 2015 by Nourish, an imprint of
Watkins Media Limited
19 Cecil Court
London, WC2N 4HE

enquiries@nourishbooks.com

Publisher: Grace Cheetham
Managing Editor: Rebecca Woods
Editor: Jan Cutler
Managing Designer: Suzanne Tuhrim
Commissioned Photography: Toby Scott
Food Stylist: Jayne Cross
Prop Stylist: Lucy Harvey
Production: Uzma Taj

A CIP record for this book is available from the
British Library

ISBN: 978-1-84899-225-2

10 9 8 7 6 5 4 3 2 1

Typeset in Rockwell
Colour reproduction by PDQ UK
Printed in China

Publisher's Note
While every care has been taken in compiling the
recipes for this book, Watkins Media Limited, or any
other persons who have been involved in working on
this publication, cannot accept responsibility for any
errors or omissions, inadvertent or not, that may be
found in the recipes or text, nor for any problems that
may arise as a result of preparing one of these recipes.
If you are pregnant or breastfeeding or have any
special dietary requirements or medical conditions, it
is advisable to consult a medical professional before
following any of the recipes contained in this book.

Notes on the Recipes
All recipes serve 1
Unless otherwise stated:
• Use medium fruit and vegetables
• Fruit and vegetables are unpeeled
• Use fresh ingredients, including herbs and spices
• Use organic ingredients where possible
• Do not mix metric and imperial measurements
• 1 tsp = 5ml   1 tbsp = 15ml   1 cup = 250ml

The nutrition symbols refer to the recipes only, not
including ingredient alternatives, optional ingredients
or serving suggestions. Peanuts, pine nuts and coconut
have been classed as nuts. Coconut sugar has been
treated as a nut-free ingredient as it is derived from
the sap rather than the nut of the coconut palm.

nourishbooks.com

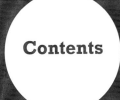

Contents

Key to Symbols

G Gluten-free
D Dairy-free
S Soya-free
N Nut-free
SE Seed-free
CI Citrus-free
V Suitable for vegans

Supercharge Your Life

For optimum health and well-being we know we need to nourish our bodies carefully, but what can we do to take our energy and vitality to a new level? How can we restore our body to the best of health and feel rejuvenated and refreshed? The answer lies in supercharging our day with foods that possess extra-powerful nutritional qualities. The easiest way to maximize your intake of these foods is through ultra-nourishing juices and smoothies. In this unique book I will show you how to revolutionize your diet by including a wide range of natural, supercharged ingredients through a collection of gorgeous, health-giving juices and smoothies, each one designed to address specific aspects of health and well-being.

The powerful foods I am going to introduce to you (that I call supercharged ingredients) will nourish your body, restoring it to a balanced and healthy state. In this way the body can function physically, emotionally and spiritually at its peak. Your energy levels will be boosted and you can enjoy vibrant and sustained health.

Each supercharged ingredient is a natural food, but it contains high concentrations of nutrients so that when you add just a small amount to a juice or smoothie it intensifies the benefits of the other fresh ingredients. There are supercharged foods to help you whether you're aiming to maintain a healthy weight, or to energize your body, boost mental and physical performance, feel radiant or support your immune system. If you include one of my supercharged juices or smoothies daily, this is all you'll need to kick-start your health. And, as you enjoy the benefits, you will feel inspired to make further lasting changes to your diet and lifestyle to improve how you feel.

I have been designing supercharged drinks like these for my clients for years and have repeatedly found that people benefit from taking them regularly. There is no need to worry about creating your own blends, because I have done all the hard work for you by devising the best combinations of fresh and supercharged foods to bring results and to taste amazing.

The simple ways to make a difference

Supercharged juices and smoothies are a surprisingly easy and satisfying way to reboot your health. Juices are gentle on the digestive system and readily assimilated by the body. The juice combinations in this book use a wide range of vegetables with some fruits, making a blend that will optimize the nutritional content of the drink without drastically upsetting blood sugar levels – essential for good health and maintaining a healthy weight.

For something more substantial, reach for your blender and whizz up one of my supercharged smoothies. Packed with soluble fibre, the smoothies will help you feel fuller for longer, providing a steady release of energy to fuel your day. They are ideal as a nourishing meal in a glass, a rejuvenating snack, post-workout fuel or a delicious and energizing treat.

Greater power from smaller doses

The recipes in this book have been developed using over 40 supercharged ingredients, plus fruit, vegetables, nuts and seeds. Many of these foods work synergistically in the body to provide optimum nourishment. My focus is on using whole foods and colourful, nutrient-rich ingredients – preferably organic – to maximize the health benefits of each drink. You need only include small amounts of the supercharged foods to have noticeable beneficial effects, because they are incredibly nutrient dense. Calorie per calorie they contain a vast quantity of concentrated beneficial nutrients to support good health compared to fresh and, especially, processed foods, which are high in calories yet devoid of nutrients.

Supercharged foods also contain a broad spectrum of vitamins, minerals and phytochemicals (natural chemicals with antioxidant properties that are found in plants). These include everyday foods (such as blueberries and kale) or less familiar foods that are available as extracts or powders (such as maca and chaga). Antioxidants found in many of the supercharged ingredients are compounds that protect the body's cells from damage by molecules known as free radicals. No matter how healthy your lifestyle is, every cell in your body is constantly bombarded by harmful chemicals. Free radicals are the chemical by-products of your body's own metabolism as well as being created from environmental toxins. Excess free radicals are a problem, because they attack the body, damaging key cellular molecules such as DNA. By protecting the body's cells from free radicals, antioxidants play a role in preventing the development of chronic diseases, such as heart disease and cancer, and help to slow ageing.

Many of these ingredients are also 'functional foods' – foods that support a particular function in the body. It is well documented, for example, that the herb maca is an adrenal adaptogen, which means that it helps the body to handle stress and to cope with stressful events.

Powerful foods from the past

Supercharged ingredients are not a new fad. In fact, many have been eaten by indigenous cultures for thousands of years and have a long history of therapeutic use. Chia seeds are one example. They have been enjoyed for centuries by cultures throughout Central America. Known as 'the running food', chia seeds and water were the main ingredients that fuelled Aztec warriors in their conquests. Today, we might think of them as a new discovery, but these foods were once everyday staples.

How to use this book

First, read the basics on the next page. The juices and smoothies are divided into chapters of fruit-based juices, vegetable-based juices, light and fruity smoothies, and richer, creamier blends. At the back of the book you will find an at-a-glance illustrated list of all the drinks with a star rating for each of the following benefits: weight loss; cleansing; radiance (anti-ageing); energy; immune health; brain health and stress. On page 9 you will find a guide to the key health categories included under each symbol.

If you suffer with blood-sugar imbalances, you should focus on vegetable-based juices and opt for the creamy smoothies where the protein and healthy fats will help to slow down the release of glucose into the bloodstream.

Many people find that their cravings for sugary, processed foods diminish and they gain a greater sense of vitality and rejuvenation in their lives. That's the power of supercharged foods!

Supercharged Basics

There are just a few basics to think about before you start, then you can begin to plan which juices and smoothies you would like to make. On the opposite page you will find the categories of health benefits that the drinks cover, and these are given a star rating in the at-a-glance section, The Quick Look, starting on page 150. Or you might like to begin with a detox weekend.

How much should you drink?
Each juice or smoothie is designed to serve one person. The recipes in this book can be used as a quick, nutritious meal alternative, an accompaniment to a meal or an energizing snack. They are also ideal for those times when you don't feel like eating; for example, during recovery from illness or when time is short.

They can form the basis of a juice or smoothie detox or a supercharged weekend blitz (page 23). Many are ideal pre- and post-workout, making them perfect for athletes or those wanting to get the most out of their training. You will also find some great ideas for anyone who is reluctant to eat more vegetables. With smoothies, you can sneak in a whole range of goodness – try the Chocolate Hazelnut Cauliflower Cream (page 114) and you'll see what I mean.

I recommend that you drink one of the drinks each day depending on your activity levels and body requirements. To help reduce your sugar intake, aim for more vegetable juices than those based on fruit. I also recommend that you focus on vegetable-based and green juices or smoothies based on protein for breakfast to avoid blood sugar imbalances first thing in the morning.

If you suffer with bacterial overgrowth or gut dysbiosis, I recommend that you avoid fruit-based juices and opt instead for vegetable-based juices or smoothies containing a higher fat and/or protein content. This is because sugars provide food for harmful microbes, contributing to a greater imbalance between beneficial and harmful bacteria as well as making a more suitable environment for yeasts and parasites.

What equipment will you need?
You will need a good-quality juicer to enable you to extract the greatest amount of nutrients from your fruit and vegetables. The cheaper juicers are not as effective at juicing leafy greens and soft fruits, which are included in many of the juices in this book, so it's worth looking around for a good one at a reasonable price. A masticating juicer is pricey but worth considering. To make citrus juices, a manual or electric citrus juicer is also useful but not essential.

To make smoothies, a high-speed blender is ideal. These blenders can also blend or crush ice, nuts and seeds and will create a smooth texture in seconds.

The only other pieces of equipment you will need are chopping boards, a sharp knife, measuring spoons and ice-cube trays – so that you can create chilled and slushy smoothies.

Choose the healthiest foods
Buy fresh fruit and vegetables and go for organic if you can. In the pantry section starting on page 10 you will find a list of the supercharged ingredients, which will mostly be available from

your supermarket or high-street health shop. In the recipes I have given a more easily available alternative, or made optional, those ingredients that need to be bought online.

Use the pantry section (starting on page 10) and the drinks index, The Quick Look (starting on page 150), to help you decide which foods to stock up on.

Extra benefits from liquids and thickeners

A range of liquids are used in this book to form the bases of the juices and smoothies, and many add health benefits as well as producing a variety of consistencies. Juices mainly use only the liquid from the fruits or vegetables – the pulp being discarded. But they can also include teas or coconut water with perhaps a little omega oil blend or aloe vera juice.

Smoothies use the whole fruit or vegetable. Many also include other liquids, as for the juices, or crushed ice. Nuts and seeds, and the milks made from them, can be added to make a thicker, more sustaining drink.

The Ultimate Smoothies, ideal for any time, are light drinks using smaller quantities of thickening agents such as nuts or seeds. The Creamy Smoothies, in contrast, use a range of foods, including yogurt and kefir – both dairy and coconut – oats, coconut flakes, protein powders and thick coconut milk. Some can be taken as a meal replacement. See page 22 for more about health-enhancing fermented drinks.

Use the symbols to make your choices

On pages 150–57 you will find a star rating for each recipe under the following benefits. Choose the recipe that has the highest star rating for the benefit you are aiming for.

W: Weight loss These smoothies and juices can help assist weight loss and fat burning. They are graded as: 5 stars (200 calories or less) – best for weight loss; 4 stars (201–250 calories); 3 stars (251–300 calories).

C: Cleansing The drinks in this category contain cleansing ingredients to help support the detoxification system and the removal of toxins from the body. They are also soothing to the digestive system or support digestive function.

R: Radiance A number of well-known 'beauty nutrients' – such as healthy fats, protein and antioxidants – are included in these juices and smoothies to support glowing skin, nails and hair. This category includes nutrients that have anti-ageing properties, helping you to look radiant and youthful.

E: Energy These juices and smoothies are designed to boost performance and energy levels. They are useful for balancing blood sugar and also contain nutrients to enhance cell health and mitochondrial function (generating energy for cells), as well as for sustained energy. Many also contain nutrients to enhance muscle mass.

I: Immune boost The nutrients in these drinks have been shown to support the body's immune system. Ingredients with anti-microbial and anti-viral properties are also included.

B: Brain health and stress These juices and smoothies contain nutrients required for brain and cognitive health. They include vitamins, minerals, healthy fats and antioxidants essential for optimal brain function.

The Supercharged Food Pantry

The potential list of supercharged foods is vast, so I have selected the more widely available superstars for this book. Many are readily available in your local supermarket or high-street health shop whereas others can be bought online.

Algae

This powerful category of ingredients includes spirulina and chlorella. Algae are single-celled organisms and one of the oldest life forms we know. They are often referred to as a near-perfect food with an exceptionally high chlorophyll content, which is one of the reasons for their powerful cleansing and restorative properties. Chlorophyll assists the body in processing more oxygen, promoting the growth and repair of tissues. (Although you should avoid algae supplements if you suffer with an iodine allergy.) Because of the potent detoxifying properties of chlorella and spirulina, I recommend that you start with a low dose and gradually build up. You can also spread the dose throughout the day. Start with ¼ teaspoon and, if you like, you can build up to 1 teaspoon. To avoid the risk of contamination from unclean sea water, choose organic algae from a reputable source.

Chlorella is a single-celled freshwater algae with a hard outer cell wall that needs to be broken down by a manufacturing process so that the body can absorb it adequately. Chlorella is particularly effective in eliminating toxins and heavy metals, such as mercury, from the body and is taken for its cleansing action on the bowel and other elimination organs. It also gives protection to the liver, helping to promote cleansing throughout the body. It contains what is known as the chlorella growth factor, which has been shown to increase the rate of tissue growth and repair, boost immune health and improve digestion. Chlorella is made up of 50 per cent complete protein. It is also abundant in vitamins and minerals, including iron and B vitamins needed for energy production. Buy as a powder or tablets. Always choose cracked-cell-wall chlorella to ensure it is digestible. See algae introduction for dosage recommendations.

Spirulina is a type of blue-green algae from warm, fresh water springs. It is many thousands of years older than chlorella and does not possess the hard cell wall. This nutrient-dense food is used to treat a wide range of ailments, including arsenic poisoning, Candida overgrowth and allergic rhinitis. It has also been seen to potentially lower stroke and cancer risk. Spirulina has immune-supporting properties, as well as helping to lower blood pressure and normalize healthy cholesterol. In addition, it is high in protein – containing 65–71 per cent complete protein compared to beef (at 22 per cent), and lentils (at 26 per cent).

Although spirulina is taken in small quantities, its high protein content will make a contribution to your overall intake. It is also an excellent source of vital amino acids and minerals, which are easily assimilated by the body. It has a cleansing effect on the body and is a powerful detoxifier. Buy as a powder or tablets. Spirulina is darker in colour and has a stronger flavour than chlorella, but you can easily add it to strong-tasting juices and smoothies, and it works particularly well in creamy drinks. See algae introduction for dosage recommendations.

Bee products

Bee pollen is the food of the young bee and is considered to be one of nature's most nourishing foods. It is about 40 per cent protein, half of which is in the form of free amino acids that are used directly by the body. This highly assimilable protein is a great strength builder and brain food. Bee pollen is rich in energizing B vitamins, vitamin C and co-enzymes as well as magnesium, calcium, copper, iron, silica, sulphur and manganese. Buy as granules.

Honey Raw and, particularly, manuka honey are rich in digestive-supporting enzymes. Honey is a powerful immune supporter with anti-microbial properties and is rich in antioxidants. As a sweetener, use only in small amounts.

Propolis is a substance collected by honey bees and used as a sealant in their hive. It contains essential oils, waxes and bioflavonoids. Buy as capsules.

Berries and fruit

Blueberries, bilberries, raspberries, straw-berries, blackberries, and so on, are well known for their superb array of nutrients. They are rich in vitamin C, but much of their health-giving properties stem from their phytonutrients, which are potent antioxidants, and many possess anti-cancer properties. Fresh berries are used in juices, although for smoothies you can also use frozen berries. You can also buy individual and mixed superfood berry powders.

Acai berry (pronounced ah-sigh-ee) is dark purple in colour and similar in size to a blueberry. It is one of the most concentrated sources of antioxidants, known as anthocyanins, which are particularly concentrated in its skin. The acai berry is high in antioxidants and is a good source of fibre, phytosterols (plant fats that help to lower LDL cholesterol), vitamins C and A and calcium, as well as healthy fats such as oleic acid (an omega-9 fat that is also found in olives) and as omega-6 essential fatty acids. As it is highly perishable, it is best to buy the freeze-dried powder or as unsweetened frozen pulp.

Amla berry Also known as Indian gooseberry, the amla berry is a rich source of vitamin C, amino acids, polyphenols, lipids and other essential oils. The berry is traditionally taken to support the digestion and liver health and to strengthen the respiratory system.

Baobab fruit Dried baobab powder is a delicious fruit extract made from the fruit of the baobab tree. It contains weight for weight more vitamin C than oranges, more iron than red meat and a rich content of the alkalizing minerals calcium, potassium and magnesium. The coconut-sized fruit has a velvety-smooth skin, and boasts a unique flavour that tastes like a blend of grapefruit, pear and vanilla.

A wonderful, revitalizing fruit, baobab is also high in malic acid, which, together with the high levels of vitamin C, boosts energy levels. Baobab powder is rich in digestive enzymes and prebiotics, which enhance the growth of probiotic bacteria in the gut, and is therefore a useful digestive aid. Its potassium, calcium and magnesium content also makes it alkalizing. Most people's bodies are acidic due to their diet and lifestyle. An alkaline environment, however, enables the cells to function better and to fight harmful diseases. By keeping the body alkaline, you keep it energized and reduce the risk of osteoporosis, muscle aches and ageing. Baobab has a slightly tart, citrusy flavour. Buy it as a freeze-dried powder.

Camu camu berry These berries are red, purple or green in colour, and similar in size to a cranberry. They have a slightly sour flavour, but this is less noticeable in the dried powder. Camu camu berries are exceptionally high in vitamin C – approximately 3,000mg per 100g/3½oz of pulp – one of the highest known of any fruit. They also contain B vitamins and trace minerals such as potassium, iron and calcium. The berry extracts have been shown to lower inflammation and oxidative stress levels. They are rich in flavonoids, low in calories and high in fibre, and may be helpful for supporting weight loss. Buy as a freeze-dried powder. Because of the high vitamin C content of camu camu berry, an excess may have a laxative effect. Use between ¼ and ½ teaspoon daily only.

Goji berries Also called wolfberries, goji berries are a vibrant red colour and have a deliciously intense flavour, like a cross between a cherry and a cranberry. They are nutrient-dense and surprisingly high in amino acids – with 18 amino acids present, including all the eight essential amino acids. This makes them ideal if you're looking for a natural vegan protein boost, and they are also high in vitamins and minerals including zinc, iron, copper, calcium, selenium and phosphorus. Goji berries contain antioxidants, especially the carotenoids, beta-carotene and zeaxanthin. Buy them as the dried berries. Powder and juice are also available.

Incan berries Also known as golden berries or cape gooseberries, fresh incan berries resemble a small yellow-orange cherry surrounded with papery husks resembling a Chinese lantern. The berries are sun-dried, enhancing their robust, citrus-like slightly sweet–sour flavour. They contain vitamins A and C, and many B vitamins, and are also high in bioflavonoids, which aid the absorption of vitamin C and help to lower inflammation in the body as well as strengthening the immune system. Buy incan berries sun-dried. They add a subtle citrus tang when blended in a smoothie.

Lucuma The delicious Peruvian lucuma fruit is prepared as a powder and sold as a natural sweetener. It has a maple-syrup flavour, adding sweetness to drinks and puddings. Lucuma contains a variety of nutrients, including vitamins, minerals and fibre, such as beta-carotene, vitamins B1, B2, B3, B5 and niacin as well as the minerals iron, potassium, calcium and phosphorus. Buy as a powder. This natural sweetener is low on the glycaemic index and has less impact on blood sugar levels than sugar.

Maqui berry has incredibly high antioxidant levels. Studies have found it to have one of the highest ORAC scores of any plant (the ORAC – oxygen radical absorbance capacities – score is a way of measuring antioxidant properties).

Topping blueberries, pomegranate and acai berries, the maqui berry contains 27,600 ORAC units per 100g/3½oz. The healing power of these antioxidants comes from the berry's ability to fight off cell-damaging free radicals, rejuvenating the body, slowing down ageing and enhancing energy levels. With powerful anti-inflammatory properties, the berry may be useful for combating chronic diseases as well as easing sore joints, aching muscles and swelling. Maqui berries have high amounts of vitamin C plus the minerals calcium and potassium. Buy maqui berries as a freeze-dried powder.

Mulberry Sun-dried mulberries have a slightly crunchy, yet wonderfully sweet, flavour. As fresh mulberries have a short shelf life, they are commonly sun-dried. They are renowned for their high antioxidant levels including phenolic flavonoid phytochemicals called anthocyanins, known for their antioxidant, anti-inflammatory, anti-microbial and anti-cancer activities, and resveratrol, known for its anti-ageing properties.

Resveratrol is a potent antioxidant to help combat inflammation, protecting the body against free-radical damage, which can lead to the development of diseases. Mulberries are an excellent source of vitamin C as well as iron, calcium, fibre, B vitamins and vitamins C and K. They are high in protein: 40g/1½oz dried mulberries contains about 4g protein. Buy the white or red berries sun-dried.

Pomegranates are exceptionally rich in vitamin C and high in polyphenols, including ellagic acid, which has been shown to help inhibit cancer cell growth. The array of antioxidants present has also been shown to support cardiovascular health. Buy pomegranate as the fresh fruit, freeze-dried powder and juice.

Sea buckthorn berries are rich in vitamins C and E, the minerals iron, chromium and manganese, amino acids, antioxidants and essential fatty acids. Buy as a juice.

Cacao

Raw, nutrient-rich unsweetened cacao powder, which is high in antioxidant flavonols, is very different from the common commercial cocoa drinks, which are high in sugar and lower in antioxidant content. Cacao is extracted from cacao beans from the fruit of the cacao tree. Loaded with antioxidants, cacao is also an excellent source of minerals including magnesium, iron, chromium, manganese, zinc and copper. It is one of the richest food sources of magnesium, which helps to relax the muscles, relieve stress and relax the heart and cardiovascular system. Cacao also contains the amino acid tryptophan, which enhances relaxation and promotes better sleep, and phenylethylamine (PEA), which has a positive effect on mood. Buy raw cacao powder, which is milder in flavour than commercial cocoa powder, and cacao nibs, which are slightly bitter and have a strong chocolate flavour. Cacao butter and paste are also available but not used in this book.

Coconut water

Sweet coconut water is refreshing added to juices and smoothies and is rich in all the beneficial electrolytes. Buy in cartons.

Dried roots, grasses, leaves and plants

Carob, technically a legume, is a naturally sweet bean-like pod. It is rich in fibre, B vitamins, vitamin E and antioxidants. The sweet, dried pods are powdered. Carob is good as an aid to digestive health. It is also useful as a chocolate substitute. Buy as a powder.

Ginkgo biloba The leaves are rich in flavonoids and terpenoids that help protect the nerves, heart muscle, blood vessels and retina from damage as well as aiding blood flow by dilating the blood vessels. It is commonly used to improve cognitive function, eyesight and circulation. Buy as a tea, tincture or powder.

Green coffee The extract derived from young green coffee beans is rich in chlorogenic acid, an antioxidant that may help with blood sugar and weight loss. Buy as a powder.

Green and matcha green tea Although black and green tea come from the same plant, green tea is less processed and therefore provides more antioxidant polyphenols, notably a catechin called epigallocatechin-3-gallate (EGCG), which is believed to be responsible for most of the health benefits. Matcha is the finely ground green tea leaves. It is a concentrated form of the tea and contains 137 times the antioxidants of regular green tea. Its rich supply of polyphenols may help green tea to protect the skin from damage, if drunk regularly.

Green tea also stimulates thermogenesis, a process that helps to raise your daily energy expenditure, increasing the use of fatty acids by the liver and muscle cells as an energy source. This is why some studies have suggested that it can promote weight loss. Green tea drinkers also appear to have a lower risk of a wide range of diseases, from bacterial or viral infections to chronic degenerative conditions including cancer and osteoporosis. Green tea contains the amino acid L-theanine, which stimulates the production of alpha brain waves to create a state of calmness and mental alertness. Buy as a powder.

Maca Also known as Peruvian ginseng, maca is regarded as an energy tonic in South America. It has been used medicinally for centuries as an adaptogen, because it has the ability to help the body adjust to stress, build up resistance to disease and support immunity. It is also useful for athletes or anyone struggling with low energy.

Maca is well supplied with antioxidants, vitamins and minerals, including calcium, magnesium and iron, vitamin C and energizing B vitamins (B1, B2, B6 and B12). It contains about 60 per cent carbohydrates, 10 per cent protein, 8.5 per cent fibre and 2.2 per cent fats, including healthy fatty acids. But the health benefits of maca appear to be mostly related to its effect on the adrenal glands and the endocrine system. Maca appears to work directly on the hypothalamus and pituitary glands, which are the 'master glands' of the body, whose role is to regulate the other glands.

Maca also appears to help balance sex hormone levels for both men and women. It may bring relief to premenstrual syndrome (PMS) sufferers and may improve libido and sexual function. It may also help alleviate menopausal symptoms such as hot flushes and night sweats. Maca has a nutty, light flavour with a slight butterscotch edge. Buy as a powder.

Moringa leaf The moringa is a rapidly growing tree (also known as the horseradish tree, drumstick tree and benzolive tree). Various parts of the plant can be used: the flower nectar as a form of honey; the oil for cooking and in cosmetics; the seeds, which are eaten green, roasted, powdered and steeped for tea or used in curries; and the leaves. Traditionally, moringa leaf has been used to lower inflammation, aid detoxification, as an antibiotic and for its anti-cancer properties. Moringa leaf contains a wealth of amino acids including all the essential amino acids, making it a useful source of protein. It is also renowned for its high chlorophyll content. Chlorophyll, the green pigment of plants, is alkalizing, cleansing and energizing, and is thought to strengthen the immune system.

Moringa is packed with antioxidants, including carotenoids and polyphenols, and vitamins, notably the B vitamins and vitamins A, C, E and K. It is high in calcium – just 5g (1 teaspoon) of the leaf powder contains 100mg. It is also a good source of magnesium, potassium, iron and sulphur. The oil is rich in oleic acid (omega-9). The leaves are often steeped in hot water to make a tea. Buy as a powder or as an oil extracted from the seeds of the plant.

Purple corn is high in antioxidants including anthocyanin. Buy as a powder.

Sprouted grasses and seeds, such as wheatgrass, sunflower sprouts, alfalfa sprouts, pea sprouts, broccoli sprouts and barley grass, are well known for their cleansing and energizing properties. Wheatgrass's popularity may be due to its exceptionally high chlorophyll content.

Sprouted grasses and seeds are alkalizing and rich in enzymes to support digestion and the absorption of nutrients. The high chlorophyll content helps to oxygenate and cleanse the blood while supporting digestive health. They are also well supplied with antioxidants and help to protect the body from damaging free radicals and toxins.

Wheatgrass has a mild, clean flavour. It is also a great source of vitamins and minerals, including the B vitamins and vitamins A and E, and the minerals calcium, phosphorus, sodium, potassium, magnesium, iron and zinc. It contains amino acids in a form that is easily absorbed by the body and is considered to have immune-supporting and anti-microbial properties.

Sprouted seeds are equally powerful. During sprouting, minerals, such as calcium and magnesium, bind to protein, making them more bio-available. In addition, the quality of the protein improves when the seeds are sprouted. The content of vitamins and essential fatty acids also increase dramatically during the sprouting process. These incredible supercharged foods help to support cell regeneration, making them potent anti-ageing and rejuvenating foods.

Fats and oils

Don't be fooled into thinking that fat is bad for you. Fat is an essential macronutrient that feeds the body and brain. The right types of fats in the correct proportions are important for lowering inflammation in the body, providing sustained energy, maintaining healthy cell membranes and the myelin sheaths (which protect the nervous system) and for forming the building blocks of hormones, which influence many biological processes throughout the body.

Coconut oil provides richness to smoothies. It contains saturated fats and is predominately rich in medium-chain triglycerides, which sustain energy levels, as they are readily utilized by the body as a fuel. It is ideal for adding to smoothies before workouts, for example. It also contains lauric acid and caprylic acid, which support immune health and possess anti-microbial properties. Buy in tubs.

Lecithin granules Made from soya or sunflower seeds, lecithin contains a naturally occurring mixture of phospholipids. The phospholipid content also contains the beneficial nutrients phosphorus, choline, inositol and glycerol. Lecithin is present in the body's cell membranes. It is particularly important for brain health and the health of the myelin sheaths that function as membranes for nerve cells. A spoonful of lecithin granules added to a smoothie or juice will give it a delicious creamy texture.

Omega-rich oils The range of oils providing the essential fatty acids omega-3 and -6 include flaxseed, chia seed and hempseed oil as well as omega-blended oils. Choose an organic cold-pressed oil for drizzling into smoothies and juices. The oils are vulnerable to damage from heat and light and are best stored in the fridge.

Fermented drinks

Kefir, kombucha and yogurt are fermented liquids, which are included in some recipes for their health benefits, particularly for supporting the digestive system and to boost immune health.

Kefir The cultured food, kefir, is rich in amino acids, enzymes, calcium, magnesium, phosphorus and B vitamins. It contains several major strains of friendly bacteria (*Lactobacillus caucasus*, Leuconostoc, Acetobacter species, and Streptococcus species) as well as beneficial yeasts, which can dramatically improve digestive function and immunity. To get the full benefit, take kefir daily (but see note below). It is made with kefir 'grains' – the mother culture. It can be made with cow's milk, sheep's milk, soya milk, coconut or nut milk. You can also make water kefir using water grains. Kefir can be made at home or purchased in health shops or online.

Kombucha is made from sweetened tea that's been fermented by a colony of bacteria and yeast (known as SCOBY). It is rich in many of the enzymes your body produces for digestion and it aids cleansing and supports liver health. Kombucha contains glucosamines, which are beneficial for cartilage structure and for preventing arthritis. It is also antioxidant rich and good for immune health. You can buy kombucha online or make your own using a SCOBY starter and any tea that you prefer for the base.

Note If you suffer with diabetes or blood sugar imbalances, it is recommended to avoid drinking kombucha or water kefir due to their sugar content. Milk or coconut kefir would be suitable, however. It is best to start slowly when taking fermented drinks to allow your body time to adjust. Start with just 4 tablespoonfuls daily or every other day for the first week.

On page 22 you will find recipes for making kombucha and kefir at home.

Medicinal mushrooms

Each medicinal mushroom possesses its own unique health-giving polysaccharides and medicinal properties. All are particularly known for their immune-supporting properties as well as improving energy, endurance and vitality. When different medicinal mushrooms are combined and consumed, the following benefits may be present. They contain a range of health-giving compounds such as mannose, which is known for its anti-microbial and anti-viral action, especially useful for urinary tract infections. They also contain a range of phytonutrients, which are understood to help slow down the ageing process. Buy medicinal mushrooms as a loose powder, or powdered in capsules, which can be opened up and tipped into drinks. They are also sometimes available as a mixed formula.

Chaga is used as an overall health tonic. It has strong immune-enhancing and anti-viral properties and high levels of antioxidants. It is often viewed as a longevity tonic and is also traditionally used for treating inflammatory conditions such as ulcers and colitis. Chaga contains a range of active ingredients: sterols, triterpenes, saponins and polysaccharides. It is an excellent choice for boosting immune health.

Cordyceps is a mushroom that can be used as a tonic herb, strengthening kidney health and promoting lung and vascular health.

Maitake is best known for its ability to detoxify carcinogens, through the beta glucan polysaccharides it contains, which have been found to promote natural cell growth and improve immune function. It is also useful in protecting the liver and aiding digestion as well as fighting bacterial and viral infections.

Reishi is a 'tonic herb', because of its ability to modulate immune function, and to promote longevity and health. It is an adaptogenic herb, helping the body to maintain balance.

Sea vegetables

Typically referred to as seaweeds, nourishing sea vegetables – kombu/kelp, wakame, arame and nori – contain a wealth of nutrients often lacking in people's diets. One tablespoon of dried sea vegetable will contain between 0.5mg and 3mg of iron, together with vitamin C, which increases the absorption of iron. Sea vegetables are high in iodine, which is essential for healthy thyroid function and metabolism, and have anti-inflammatory and anti-viral properties. When selecting sea vegetables, check that they come from certified clean water sources. Opt for organic where possible. Buy as a powder, granules or flakes, or buy nori in sheets.

Seeds

Many seeds possess extremely high levels of life-giving nutrients, including protein, fats, minerals and fibre. Adding seeds or a seed butter to a drink can help to thicken the liquid as well as providing a creamy texture. Keep a range of seeds in your pantry. As well as the super-seeds below, stock up on nutrient-rich sunflower, pumpkin and sesame seeds.

Chia The tiny black chia seed is a powerhouse of nutrition. The seeds are prized for their amazingly high omega-3 content, which is beneficial for brain function, lowering inflammation and for cardiovascular health, and as a beauty food. They are also rich in antioxidants, which help to protect the vulnerable omega-3 fats from deterioration. Their high soluble-fibre content means that they absorb water readily, plumping up and thickening a liquid to form a gel. This attribute supports digestive health, easing constipation, and as the seeds swell in the stomach they create a feeling of fullness, making them ideal for weight loss and cleansing. Nearly 20 per cent of your daily calcium need is contained in just 30g/1oz chia seeds and they also contain 4g protein and 11g fibre. Buy as the whole seed (black or white), ground, or sprouted and ground. Their high omega-3 fat content can be destroyed by heat and light, so it is best to store them in the fridge.

Flaxseed is a great source of essential omega-3, -6 and -9 fats. It is also one of the best food sources of lignans – unique fibre-related polyphenols that provide the body with antioxidant benefits and act as phytoestrogens, which help to balance hormone levels. The antioxidant levels, together with the high-fibre content of flaxseed, make it useful for stabilizing blood sugar, which helps to control appetite and cravings for sugary foods. It also has a high mucilage content making the water-soluble, gel-forming fibre soothing for the digestive tract. With its good source of manganese and magnesium, flaxseed is useful for sustaining energy levels too. Flaxseed helps to thicken juices and smoothies. Buy as the whole seed, ground seed, sprouted and ground, and the oil.

Hemp seeds and their oil are an excellent source of essential fatty acids. Linoleic acid, the omega-6 essential fatty acid, accounts for about two-thirds of the essential fatty acids found in hemp seeds. The other third comes from the omega-3 fatty acid, alpha-linolenic acid (ALA), that forms the starting point for production of all other omega-3s in the body. Hemp is, in fact, a powerhouse of nutrition. Containing all 20 amino acids, including the essential amino acids, hemp is a fabulous protein food for vegetarians and vegans. It is rich in a range of nutrients, including the B vitamins, vitamin E, carotene, calcium and magnesium. It also provides soluble fibre to help satisfy the appetite and curb cravings. Hemp has a light, nutty flavour. Buy as shelled hemp seeds or whole seeds and hemp oil. Hemp protein powder is also available. Like other seeds rich in essential fats, it is best stored in the fridge.

Supercharged herbs

Apart from the herbs listed, there are many others with adaptogenic properties used to support the adrenal glands or as energy tonics. Buy as powders, teas, tinctures, extracts or syrups. These include liquorice, astragalus, rhodiola, ashwagandha and gynostemma. Other beneficial teas to take, especially for digestion and detoxification, include nettle and dandelion.

Aloe vera The numerous healing properties of aloe include anti-inflammatory and immune-modulating effects and cancer-protective qualities. It is useful for supporting digestive health, soothing the gut and improving the digestion of nutrients. It can also boost levels of friendly gut bacteria by providing an environment in which they can flourish, as well as reducing acidity and boosting digestive-enzyme function. It is a cleansing tonic, for radiant skin, supporting immune health and fighting microbial and viral infections, and it may help with menstruation issues. Buy juices and gels for internal use to add to juices and smoothies – made from the whole leaf extract, they do not have a laxative effect.

Cissus quadrangularis is beneficial for healthy bones, the digestion, menstruation, respiration and halting an excess of the stress hormone cortisol. Buy as a powder or tincture.

Echinacea supports immune function and is typically used for the treatment and prevention of upper respiratory tract infections, colds and flu. Buy as a tincture, powder or tea.

Ginseng products are usually used as a general tonic and adaptogen to help the body resist the daily stresses placed upon it. It is often used to improve physical and mental performance, vitality and to reduce fatigue. Its properties appear to be the result of a range of compounds present – ginsenosides, saponins, phytosterols, peptides, polysaccharides, fatty acids and polyacetylenes, as well as vitamins and minerals. There are several species of ginseng and their exact effect will be influenced by the type and amounts of ginsenosides present. They appear to help improve immune function, reduce inflammation, improve insulin sensitivity and protect the body from nerve damage, and they might have anti-cancer properties too. Panax ginseng is often chosen for its abilities to help tackle stress. American ginseng can be used to improve blood-sugar handling or to moisten the body – easing dry coughs, for example. Eleuthero ginseng, or Siberian ginseng, is an excellent energy, stress and blood tonic – great for athletes. Buy as a powder, tincture or tea.

Schizandra is a traditional herb used to enhance energy in the liver and kidneys as well as to support the memory and sexual health. Buy as a powder, a tea and a tincture.

He shou wu is widely used in Chinese tonic herbalism to prevent premature ageing by tonifying the kidney and liver functions, nourishing the blood and fortifying the muscles, tendons and bones. It is also used to enhance sexual drive, increase sperm count and to strengthen the sperm and ova. It is rich in zinc and iron. Buy as a powder and a tea.

Milk thistle is used to support the health and function of the liver. It can help to increase the flow of bile (which emulsifies fats and excretes waste from the body). Research has shown that milk thistle is able to protect the liver from the damaging effects of a variety of toxins, partly because it is a powerful antioxidant. It is also used for detoxification. Buy as a tincture or tea.

Shatavari is a form of wild asparagus that has been used for centuries to support women's health. It is often regarded as a woman's most powerful supercharged herb, traditionally used to boost fertility, improve menopausal symptoms and build healthy oestrogens in the female body. Buy as a powder, tincture or tea.

Turmeric is a culinary spice whose health benefits lie in its active ingredient, curcumin, known for its potent anti-inflammatory and antioxidant properties. Much research has been undertaken into its ability to help with autoimmune and inflammatory conditions including inflammatory bowel diseases, rheumatoid arthritis, cancer prevention and for reducing the risk of cognitive decline, including Alzheimer's. Curcumin also supports liver health and reduces cardiovascular risk. The active component is better absorbed when combined with a little black pepper and fat. Buy the fresh root or use ground turmeric.

Additional nutrients

Collagen, the most abundant protein in the body, is found in the skin, bones, ligaments, cartilage, teeth and muscles. It is essential for bone health and for building the bone matrix. Collagen powder supplements may assist the following: gut and joint health; a clearer complexion; to lower inflammation; to strengthen weak nails and thicken fine hair; to repair connective tissues for improved elasticity; to help improve circulation; and to promote wound healing. Hydrolyzed collagen is a pre-digested form of collagen, which is more easily absorbed. Buy as a powder. Also available in a liquid form.

Colostrum is the first food a mammal gives to her offspring. It is nature's most concentrated source of biologically active components. Colostrum contains over 80 per cent of the bioactive components produced in the bone marrow and circulatory system. There are over 90 known beneficial components in bovine colostrums, including immunoglobulins, transfer factors, lactoferrin, transferrin, insulin-like growth factor, fat-soluble vitamins (A, D, E and K) and protein. Colostrum is used extensively to support overall immune health and digestive health, and to facilitate healing and recovery after exercise, illness and surgery. Buy as a powder.

Glutamine is an amino acid (a building block of protein) found in the muscles of the body. Although under normal circumstances the body can manufacture sufficient for its daily requirement, there are times when glutamine becomes needed to counter physical stress, such as after surgery and during wound healing, cancer, exercise and burns. Supplementing can therefore be beneficial. Glutamine helps to promote a healthy digestive tract, support immune health and fight infection, and may also decrease sugar cravings. It is beneficial to take as a support for recovery and repair, and helping to optimize a training and exercise programme. Stress and illness can lead to a loss in muscle mass if insufficient glutamine is available, making supplements beneficial. Buy as a powder.

MSM (methylsulfonylmethane) is a naturally occurring sulphur compound normally present in small amounts in humans and in many foods, but it is rapidly depleted or lost through food processing. MSM is used to improve the health of the hair, skin and nails, for joint health and reducing inflammation in arthritic conditions. Buy as a powder.

Probiotics Beneficial bacteria (probiotics) are naturally present in the gut, and their essential role in the digestion and absorption of food makes them vital for good health. Probiotics actively synthesize the essential vitamins K2 and the B vitamins. They also help to prevent the colonization of harmful microbes such as bacteria and yeast, and help to modulate our immune health and lower inflammation. Beneficial bacteria can be easily diminished through stress, medications and a poor diet. Probiotic powders are a convenient way to increase your levels of healthy bacteria. Buy as a powder.

Protein powders These can be useful for improving the protein content of a juice or smoothie, thereby helping to stabilize blood sugar as well as supporting immune health, facilitating growth and the repair of tissues, and helping to maintain healthy body composition. A protein-rich smoothie can act as a meal replacement. They are also used for sports training and recovery, post-surgical recovery and during periods of loss of appetite, such as post-illness or during chemotherapy. The quality of protein powders varies tremendously. Buy a high-quality powder without fillers, additives

and sweeteners. Although whey protein powders contain a good bio-available source of amino acids and other components to support health, many people find dairy products difficult to digest. Other forms, such as pea protein, rice, hemp and superfood blends, may be more suitable and are readily available. If they are flavoured, look for natural flavourings only, and ideally choose an organic product.

Shilajit is a potent mineral supplement used in Ayurvedic medicine and made from a brown pitch or tar that exudes from layers of mountain rock. Shilajit contains all the organic and ionic dietary minerals, trace minerals and ultra-trace minerals. Humic and fulvic acid are present: humic acid has been demonstrated in research to be a potent anti-viral agent, whereas fulvic acid is a detoxifier. Buy as a powder.

Tocotrienols Commonly derived from rice bran, this whole food provides a natural, concentrated source of bio-available vitamin E plus other nutrients and plant-based fats. It is rich in antioxidants, B vitamins and minerals, including calcium, potassium, magnesium, phosphorus, iron, zinc, copper and iodine. Buy as a powder.

MAKING SUBSTITUTIONS

Although some supercharged foods can be expensive, just one pack will go a long way, as you will be using less than a teaspoonful in most recipes. You can simply omit some of them altogether – the drink will still taste delicious and be nutrient-rich, because all the ingredients have been chosen for their beneficial properties. In the recipes you will find suggested alternatives for the more unusual ingredients, and you can also make the following substitutions: instead of cacao powder use cocoa powder, but reduce the amount to taste, as it is normally stronger in flavour; instead of chlorella and spirulina use green superfood blends, wheatgrass powder or moringa powder; instead of dried mulberries, incan berries or goji berries, use raisins, dried cherries or dried cranberries; instead of macadamia nuts use cashew nuts.

HEALTHY PANTRY STAPLES

In addition to the key supercharged foods and the nut and seed milks below, it is worth keeping some healthy staples to add flavour and nutrition to your drinks. These include:

Coconut milk Tinned coconut milk makes a rich and nourishing base for drinks.

Dried fruits Dates, apricots, prunes, figs, and so on, are useful for adding a little sweetness to smoothies.

Frozen fruit and vegetables In addition to fresh produce, frozen fruits and vegetables are an economical choice for smoothies.

Herbs and spices Fresh herbs make a delicious and nutritious addition to juices and smoothies and contain medicinal properties. Ideally, keep pots of parsley and mint growing through the year to pick and use. Fresh spices to buy include root ginger, garlic and chillies, plus dried ground cinnamon and turmeric.

Chicory or dandelion coffee are healthy alternatives to regular coffee.

Himalayan sea salt A dash of Himalayan sea salt can help to lift the flavour of smoothies and it also provides trace minerals.

Natural sweeteners The majority of the recipes avoid any additional sweetener, but you may wish to have a range of healthier natural alternatives to hand. In addition to manuka honey, bee pollen and lucuma, the following have a lower glycaemic index than cane sugar, so they will not disrupt blood sugar levels as much: xylitol, coconut sugar, coconut syrup or stevia.

Nuts and seeds and their butters You can buy nuts and seeds in bulk and store them sealed in containers in the fridge or freezer to maximize shelf life. Store opened nut and seed butters in the fridge.

Nutritional yeast flakes Adding a spoonful of nutritional yeast flakes to savoury juices and smoothies provides a salty, cheese-like flavour. They are rich in B vitamins, minerals and protein.

MILKS, FERMENTED DRINKS AND NOURISHING ICES

Supercharge your drinks by using liquid bases and ices that possess additional health benefits.

Nut and seed milks

Below is an almond milk recipe, but you can also use cashew nuts, sunflower seeds or pumpkin seeds. Or you can also blend 2–3 tablespoons nut butter with 750ml/26fl oz/3 cups water for an instant milk. Change the flavour of the basic recipe by adding 2 dates for sweetness, a little vanilla extract or spices, such as cinnamon, or some cacao powder for a chocolate version.

Basic Nut Milk

160g/5½oz/1 cup almonds

Put the almonds in a bowl and cover with water. Leave for 4–6 hours, then drain. Put the nuts in a blender or food processor with 750ml/26fl oz/ 3 cups water (or 500ml/17fl oz/2 cups water for a thicker milk). Blend until liquid, then strain through a nut-milk bag, a fine sieve or muslin. Add up to 250ml/9fl oz/1 cup water to thin the milk, if you like. Store in the fridge for 3 days.

Making fermented drinks

When making the fermented drinks, kefir and kombucha, do not use metal equipment or utensils. Use wooden or plastic spoons, a plastic strainer and plastic or glass bowls.

Home-Made Kefir

You must use organic milk for kefir. Either use organic UHT milk or heat pasteurized milk to just below boiling point, and cool it before using.

Milk Kefir

1 sachet of milk kefir grains
1l/35fl oz/4 cups organic UHT full-fat milk or milk alternative, such as soya, coconut or nut milk

Put the kefir into a large sterilized glass jar and pour over the milk. Stir well. Cover with a lid, but do not seal, and leave to ferment in a warm place, away from direct sunlight, for at least 24 hours. The milk will separate to form the kefir liquid underneath. Strain through a sieve and reserve the grains, then start the process again. Store the kefir in the fridge for up to 4 days. If you regularly make kefir with coconut, nut or soya milk, store the grains in dairy milk between batches to enable them to feed.

Water Kefir

70g/2½oz/scant ⅓ cup caster sugar
1 sachet of water kefir grains
½ lemon
1 thin slice of fresh ginger, peeled (optional)

Put 750ml/26fl oz/3 cups filtered, boiled and cooled water (or coconut water) into a glass jar. Add the sugar and leave to dissolve. Add the remaining ingredients. Cover, but do not seal, and leave to ferment at room temperature for 24–72 hours, depending on the strength you prefer. Strain the water kefir and bottle it in smaller containers. Drink immediately or leave for a further 24 hours to continue fermenting. Re-use the kefir grains to make another batch.

Home-Made Kombucha

4–6 tea bags or 1½ tbsp loose-leaf tea
170g/6oz/¾ cup caster or granulated sugar or coconut sugar
1 packet of kombucha starter culture (SCOBY)

Put the tea bags in a large sterilized glass container and add the sugar. Pour over 750ml/26fl oz/3 cups boiling water. Stir well and leave the mixture to cool to room temperature. Add the SCOBY. Cover with a cloth or muslin and leave in a warm place for 3–14 days to brew. The liquid will become a little cloudier when ready. After 3 days, taste the brew. If it tastes fruity and not like tea, it's ready. If not, leave it for another day. Strain the mixture, but leave a little in the container with the SCOBY to make another batch. Store the brew in the fridge for up to 4 days – it will get fizzier, but it is still fine to drink.

Nourishing ices

Pour coconut water, coconut milk, nut milks or herbal teas into ice-cube trays and freeze until solid. Pop them out and store them in freezer-proof bags ready for use. You will need 4–5 ice cubes for one smoothie, or 8–10 for a slushy, frosty drink.

Your Supercharged Detox Blitz Weekend

This Blitz Weekend is an effective way to kick-start a new healthy-eating programme of supercharged foods. It is an intensive juice and smoothie weekend containing nutrient-dense drinks designed to cleanse and revitalize the body. To get the best results, start tweaking your diet, as below, the week before the juice day.

Start preparations for the detox blitz at least one or two days beforehand. Gradually cut back on known allergenic foods and stimulants including caffeine, alcohol, sugary drinks and foods, red meat, grains – particularly gluten grains (wheat, barley, rye) – and dairy foods (except kefir and yogurt, which are fermented and easier to digest). Increase your intake of water, coconut water and herbal teas, aiming for 6–8 glasses a day. If there is a smoothie or juice from the book that you prefer rather than the ones listed, adapt the plan accordingly. I have included predominately green-based juices with thicker detox smoothies for lunch and dinner to help with balancing blood sugar levels during each day.

Alternatively, you could do a juice-until-dinner day. This would involve three cleansing juices (for breakfast, lunch and in the afternoon) and then a light meal, such as poached salmon and steamed vegetables, in the evening.

To maximize your results, you could include a massage, facial, sauna or beauty treatment. You can also include some gentle exercise such as walking, yoga, a gentle swim, and so on.

Do not follow the detox if you are pregnant. If you have a chronic illness or are on long-term medication, or if you suffer with blood sugar imbalances or diabetes, speak to your health practitioner before considering a detox day.

Supercharged Blitz Weekend schedule

DAY ONE
On waking: a glass of warm water with the juice of ½ lemon

Breakfast: Electrolyte Burst (page 54)

Mid morning: a glass of water, coconut water or herbal tea

Lunch: Spinach Blend (page 61) and a glass of water

Mid afternoon: a glass of water or herbal tea and Spicy Golden Lemonade (page 32)

Dinner: Avocado Greens (page 84)

Evening Drink: herbal tea, coconut water, home-made nut milk (page 21)

DAY TWO
On waking: a glass of warm water with the juice of ½ lemon

Breakfast: Chlorophyll Wonder (page 54)

Mid morning: a glass of water, coconut water or herbal tea

Lunch: Magnesium Lift (page 94) and a glass of water

Mid afternoon: Golden Blend (page 80)

Dinner: Shamrock Shake (page 124)

Evening Drink: herbal tea, coconut water, home-made nut milk (page 21)

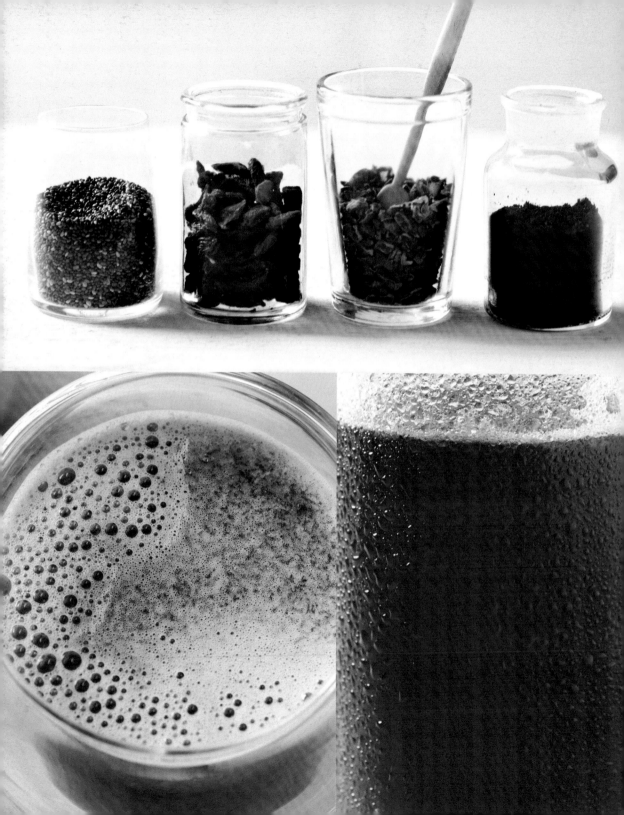

CHAPTER 1

FRUIT-BASED JUICES

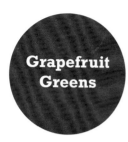

Grapefruit Greens

Pictured>

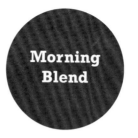

Morning Blend

2 apples
2 oranges, peeled
1cm/½in piece of root ginger, peeled
5mm/¼in piece of TURMERIC ROOT or
   a large pinch of ground TURMERIC
¼ tsp CAMU CAMU powder, or BAOBAB
   powder or ACAI BERRY powder

½ romaine or cos lettuce
1 pink grapefruit, peeled
1 apple
¼ tsp MATCHA GREEN TEA powder

Tart and tangy, with an underlying sweetness, this citrusy green juice makes a terrific morning drink. Blending in matcha green tea powder gives this juice a terrific antioxidant boost and makes it a useful weight-loss drink, because green tea has been shown to stimulate the metabolism.

Shop-bought processed orange juice is a poor substitute for the real thing. Instead, make up this zingy anti-inflammatory mix. If you can get fresh turmeric root, add this to the juicer as well, but if not, you can blend in turmeric powder at the end. Camu camu powder is a good way to boost the vitamin C level, making it ideal for improving your immunity.

Put all the ingredients, except the matcha, through an electric juicer. Transfer to a blender or food processor and add the matcha, then blend until smooth. Serve the juice immediately.

Put the apples, oranges, ginger and turmeric root (but not the ground turmeric) through an electric juicer. Transfer to a blender or food processor and add the ground turmeric, if using, and the camu camu powder, then blend until smooth. Serve the juice immediately.

(G) (D) (S) (N) (SE) (V)

(G) (D) (S) (N) (SE) (V)

Nutritional information per serving
Kcals 98 | **Protein** 3.5g
Carbohydrates 19.5g, of which sugars 19.5g
Fat 0.8g, of which saturates 0g

Nutritional information per serving
Kcals 182 | **Protein** 5.1g
Carbohydrates 62.5g, of which sugars 34.5g
Fat 0.4g, of which saturates 0g

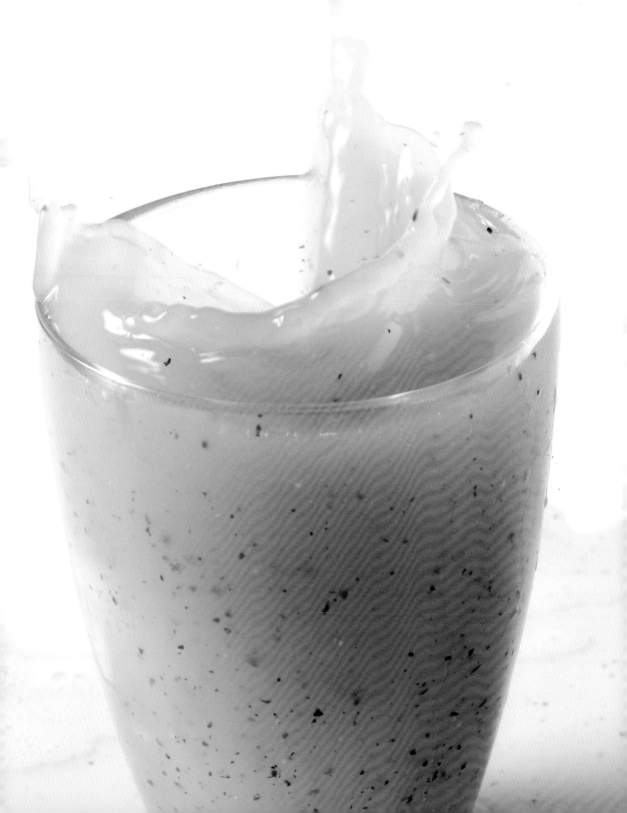

Creamy C Revitalizer

¼ pineapple, skin cut off
1 pear
2 celery sticks
1 small lemon, peeled
1cm/½in piece of root ginger, peeled
¼ tsp **BAOBAB** powder
½ tsp **PROBIOTIC** powder
1 tsp **COLOSTRUM** powder or **GLUTAMINE** powder

Give your body an immune lift with this revitalizing juice. The addition of vitamin C-rich baobab, plus probiotics and colostrum, helps nourish the immune system and support your digestion too.

Put the pineapple, pear, celery, lemon and ginger through an electric juicer, then stir in the remaining ingredients. (Alternatively, transfer to a blender or food processor and process to blend in the remaining ingredients.) Serve immediately.

Health Benefits
Colostrum is a first milk from cows produced immediately after calving. It is incredibly rich in rejuvenating nutrients: it contains immune-system properties and growth factors with potent anti-viral, anti-bacterial, anti-inflammatory and anti-parasitic properties, making it highly beneficial for those suffering with autoimmune diseases, allergies and digestive conditions. Colostrum is regularly used to boost the immune system, improve digestive health, and build and repair tissue.

Nutritional information per serving
Kcals 170 | **Protein** 4.9g
Carbohydrates 58.9g, of which sugars 29.9g
Fat 0.9g, of which saturates 0g

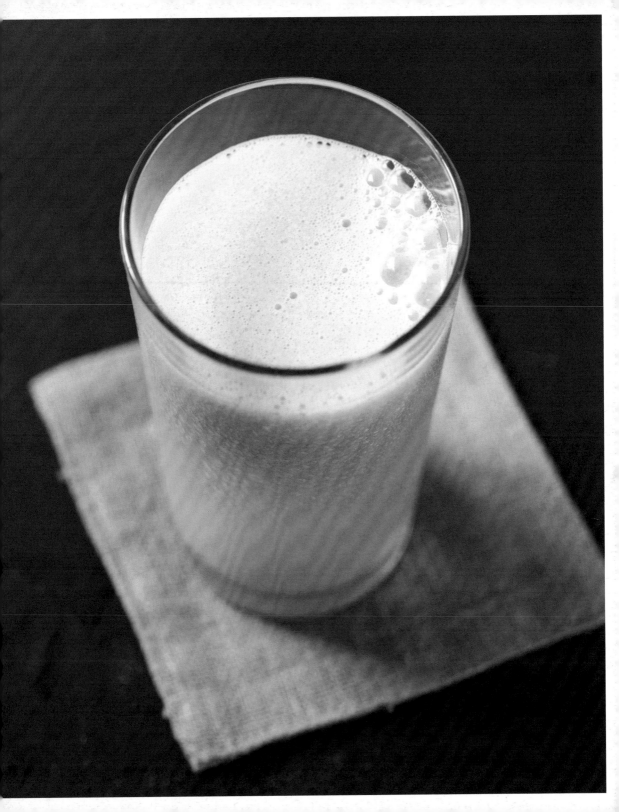

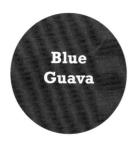

Blue Guava

1 handful of pak choi or spinach leaves
1 apple
½ pear
80g/2¾oz/½ cup blueberries
½ lemon, peeled
1 guava, peeled, or drained, tinned guava
¼ tsp GINSENG powder
COCONUT WATER, to thin as needed

Guavas are a sweet, creamy and juicy
tropical fruit with high levels of vitamin
C as well as containing vitamin A, B
vitamins and potassium, making this an
antioxidant-packed, energizing drink.
Ginseng gives it an additional kick,
which makes the juice especially useful
when you're feeling low in energy.

Put all the ingredients, except the guava,
ginseng powder and coconut water, through
an electric juicer. Transfer to a blender
or food processor and add the guava and
ginseng powder, then blend until smooth.
Add coconut water to thin the juice to your
liking. Serve immediately.

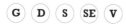

Nutritional information per serving
Kcals 106 | **Protein** 2g
Carbohydrates 24.3g, of which sugars 23.8g
Fat 0.8g, of which saturates 0g

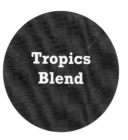

Tropics Blend

1 lime, peeled
¼ pineapple, skin cut off
1 handful of spinach
2 passion fruits, pulp and seeds only
3 lychees, peeled and pitted
1 tsp TOCOTRIENOLS or 1 tsp CHIA
    SEED OIL

Drink this sweet and creamy juice,
and dream of sunny tropical holidays,
while the antioxidant properties of the
ingredients go to work. Include the core
of the pineapple because it is rich in the
anti-inflammatory enzyme bromelain.

Put the lime, pineapple and spinach through
an electric juicer. Transfer to a blender
or food processor and add the remaining
ingredients, then blend until smooth. Serve
the juice immediately.

Ⓖ Ⓓ Ⓢ Ⓝ ⓈⒺ Ⓥ

Nutritional information per serving
Kcals 74 | **Protein** 1.9g
Carbohydrates 16.6g, of which sugars 16.6g
Fat 0.5g, of which saturates 0.1g

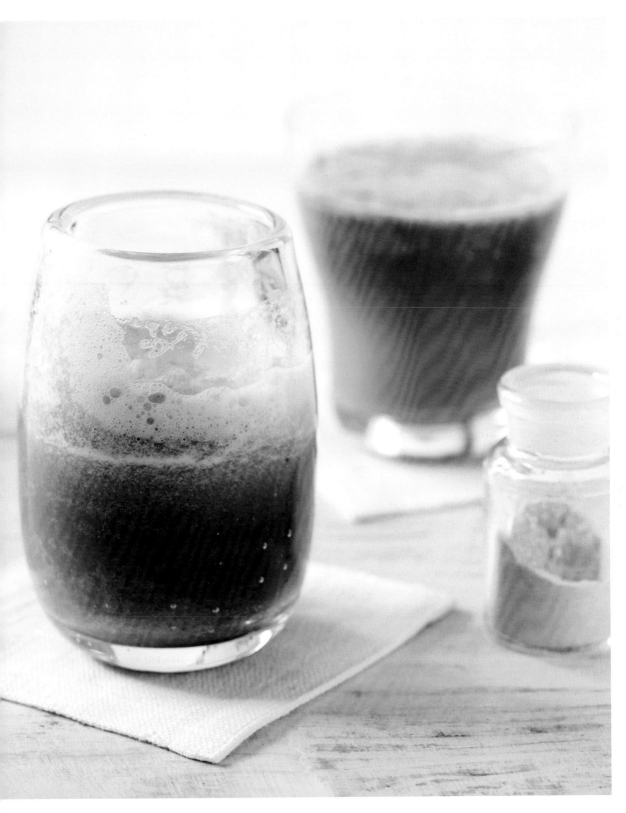

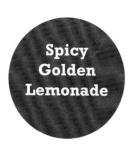

Spicy Golden Lemonade

1 lemon, peeled
2 apples
1cm/½in piece of root ginger, peeled (optional)
2 tbsp GOJI BERRIES
a pinch of cayenne pepper
¼ tsp CAMU CAMU powder, or BAOBAB powder or ACAI BERRY powder
1 tsp MANUKA or RAW HONEY (optional)
fizzy water, to serve

Give your body a makeover in the morning with this revitalizing spiced lemonade. Antioxidant-rich goji berries have skin-protective properties that can shield the skin from sun exposure. Cayenne pepper helps to stimulate the metabolism, while lemon juice is known for its digestive and cleansing properties. This drink is ideal for a detox juice cleanse.

Put the lemon, apples and ginger, if using, through an electric juicer. Add the goji berries and leave to soak for 30 minutes. Transfer to a blender or food processor and add the remaining ingredients except the fizzy water. Blend until smooth and golden in colour. Pour into a glass and top up with fizzy water. Serve immediately.

(G) (D) (S) (N) (SE) (V)

Nutritional information per serving
Kcals 219 | **Protein** 3.8g
Carbohydrates 70.1g, of which sugars 38.2g
Fat 2g, of which saturates 0g

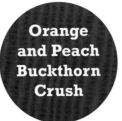

Orange and Peach Buckthorn Crush

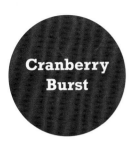

Cranberry Burst

2 handfuls of fresh or frozen cranberries
1 lime, peeled
2 oranges, peeled
1 tsp **MANUKA** or **RAW HONEY** (optional)

This slightly tart, tangy juice makes a wonderful party drink served with fizzy water – perfect for Christmas. Cranberries contain an exceptionally high content of proanthocyanidins – plant antioxidants – and are well known to help combat urinary tract infections. They also possess strong anti-inflammatory properties and may help to reduce the risk of periodontal disease (tooth decay).

Put the cranberries, lime and oranges through an electric juicer, then stir in the honey, if using. Serve immediately.

 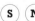 (G) (D) (S) (N) (SE) (V)

Nutritional information per serving
Kcals 138 | **Protein** 4.1g
Carbohydrates 31.4g, of which sugars 30.6g
Fat 0.5g, of which saturates 0g

1 lime, peeled
2 oranges, peeled
2 peaches, pitted and chopped
1 tsp **BEE POLLEN** or **RAW HONEY**
2 tbsp **SEA BUCKTHORN** juice (optional)
4 **COCONUT ICE CUBES** (page 22) or
    ice cubes

Cool down on hot summer days with this light juice packed with rejuvenating vitamin C and antioxidants, and blended with ice to create a refreshing slushy drink. Sea buckthorn juice possesses healing properties and, being rich in antioxidant polyphenols, it is a natural anti-ageing food.

Put the lime and oranges through an electric juicer. Transfer to a blender or food processor and add the peaches, bee pollen and sea buckthorn juice, if using. Blend until smooth. Add the ice and blend to create a slushy drink.

 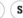 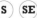 (G) (D) (S) (SE)

Nutritional information per serving
Kcals 144 | **Protein** 4.5g
Carbohydrates 30.6g, of which sugars 29.7g
Fat 0.5g, of which saturates 0.1g

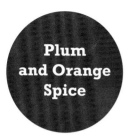

Plum and Orange Spice

3 plums, pitted
5 strawberries, stalks discarded
2 oranges, peeled
1 apple
1cm/½in piece of root ginger, peeled
1 tsp COCONUT OIL, melted

The flavour of ginger with the fruit makes this a luxurious-tasting juice. Plums and strawberries are both good sources of vitamin C, which helps to protect the body, including the brain, from free-radical damage, whereas the coconut oil nourishes the skin and brain. Strawberries are also a rich source of ellagic acid, a polyphenol shown to reduce inflammation and protect the body from cancer.

Put all the ingredients, except the oil, through an electric juicer, then stir in the oil. Serve immediately.

Nutritional information per serving
Kcals 196 | **Protein** 3.9g
Carbohydrates 39.9g, of which sugars 38.9g
Fat 3.5g, of which saturates 2.6g

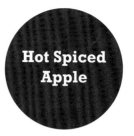

Hot Spiced Apple

3 apples
½ lime, peeled
1–2 tsp MANUKA or RAW HONEY, to taste
2 star anise
1 cinnamon stick
1cm/½in piece of root ginger, peeled and sliced
½ tsp CAMU CAMU powder, or BAOBAB powder or ACAI BERRY powder
a few drops of ECHINACEA tincture

The perfect choice for cold winter evenings – a delicious mixture of spices and honey gives this juice a comforting, aromatic flavour. A dash of echinacea provides an additional immune boost for this invigorating drink.

Put the apples and lime through an electric juicer. Pour the juice into a saucepan and add the honey and spices. Heat gently for 2 minutes, stirring frequently, then strain through a sieve. Stir in the camu camu powder and echinacea. Serve immediately.

 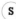

Nutritional information per serving
Kcals 143 | **Protein** 2.8g
Carbohydrates 55.1g, of which sugars 27.1g
Fat 0.3g, of which saturates 0g

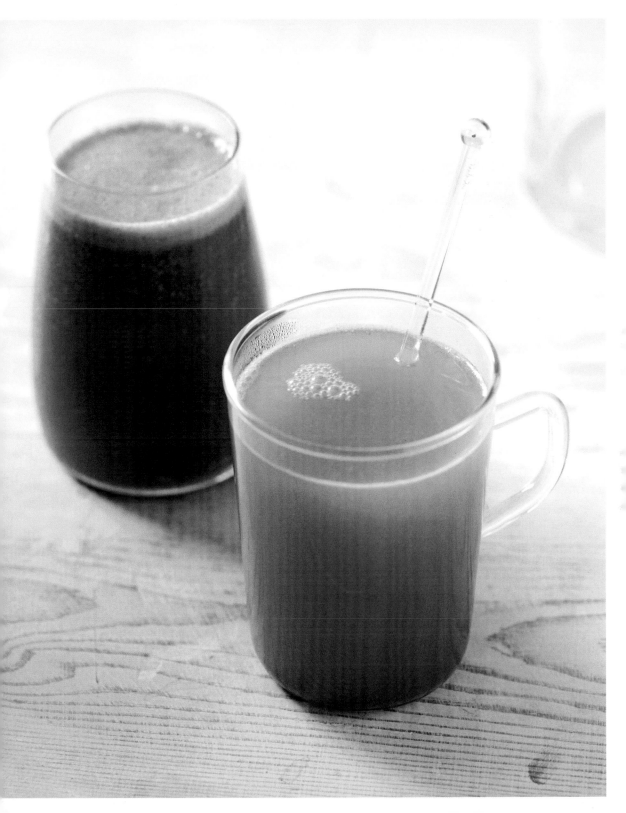

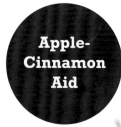

Apple-Cinnamon Aid

3 apples
1½ limes, peeled
150ml/5fl oz/scant ⅔ cup sparkling water
1 tsp **RAW** or **MANUKA HONEY**, or coconut syrup
¼ tsp ground cinnamon
4 ice cubes

Cool and deliciously refreshing, this lightly spiced fizzy apple juice is less sugary than shop-bought apple juice. You could also make it with pears instead of apples, for a change.

Put the apples and limes through an electric juicer, then stir in the water, honey and cinnamon. Serve over ice.

(G) (D) (S) (N) (SE)

Nutritional information per serving
Kcals 98 | **Protein** 1.1g
Carbohydrates 24g, of which sugars 23.6g
Fat 0.3g, of which saturates 0g

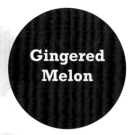

Gingered Melon

¼ watermelon
¼ cantaloupe melon
1cm/½in piece of root ginger, peeled
¼ tsp **MACA** powder

Simple, tasty and refreshing, this juice has a dash of ginger to help support the digestion and alleviate heartburn. The watermelon contains lycopene, a powerful anti-inflammatory and antioxidant, valuable for cardiovascular and bone health. A little maca powder turns this juice into a natural tonic to promote energy and ease stress.

Cut the flesh of both pieces of melon away from the peel. Discard the peel. Put all the ingredients, except the maca powder, through an electric juicer, then stir in the maca powder. Serve immediately.

(G) (D) (S) (N) (SE) (CI) (V)

Nutritional information per serving
Kcals 110 | **Protein** 2.4g
Carbohydrates 23.1g, of which sugars 22.9g
Fat 0.9g, of which saturates 0.3g

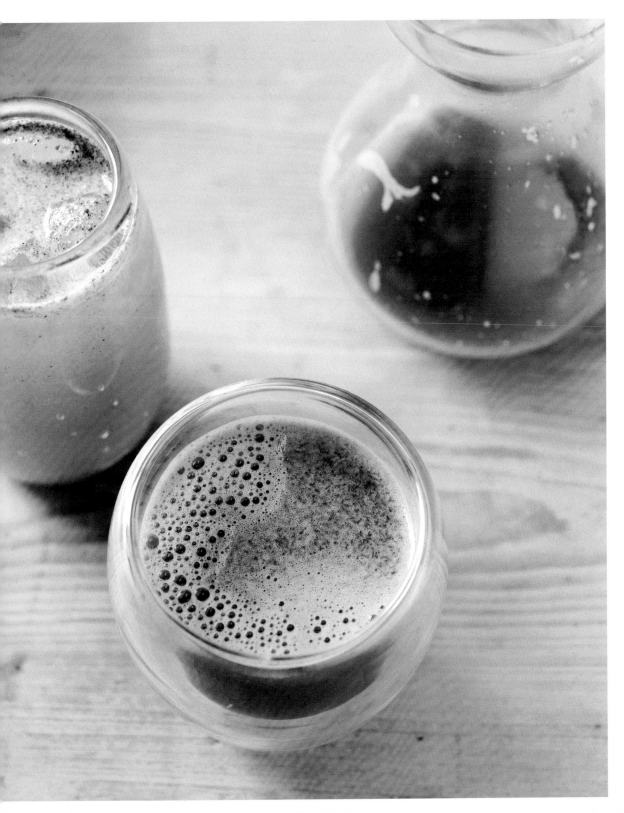

Apricot Immune

4 apricots, pitted
4 carrots
1 peach, pitted
1 orange, peeled
a few drops of ECHINACEA tincture
¼–½ tsp CHAGA powder, MEDICINAL MUSHROOM powder or MACA powder, to taste

Sip this antioxidant immune booster on those days when you are feeling under the weather. Vibrant orange in colour, this juice is rich in vitamin C, carotenoids, potassium and magnesium to boost your energy and improve stamina. Apricots also provide iron to keep you feeling vibrant, plus silicon – a wonderful hair and skin tonic.

Put the apricots, carrots, peach and orange through an electric juicer, then stir in the echinacea tincture and chaga powder. (Alternatively, transfer to a blender or food processor and process to blend in the echinacea and chaga.) Serve immediately.

Health Benefits
Chaga powder and medicinal mushrooms are potent anti-ageing immune-boosting supercharged foods. Known particularly for their cancer-fighting properties, they are also high in vital phytochemicals, nutrients and protective antioxidants, including melanin, a pigment found in the skin and the eye's retina.

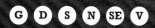

Nutritional information per serving
Kcals 159 | Protein 4.2g
Carbohydrates 36.5g, of which sugars 34.2g
Fat 0.7g, of which saturates 0.1g

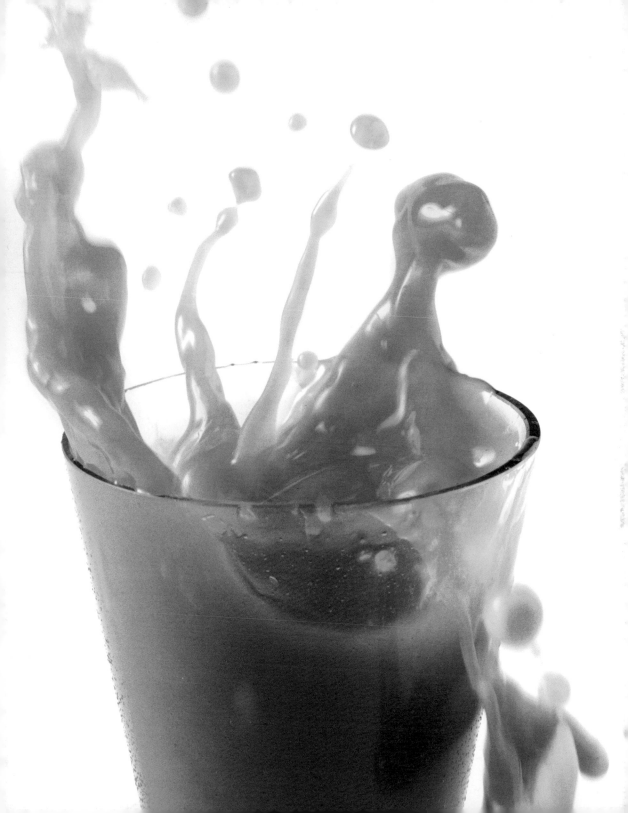

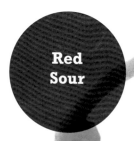

Red Sour

5 strawberries, stalks discarded
60g/2¼oz/½ cup raspberries
1 pink grapefruit, peeled
¼ papaya, peeled and deseeded
½ tsp BAOBAB power

With its abundance of antioxidants, this zingy juice is a perfect way to start the day. Pink grapefruits are a great source of lycopene, a potent antioxidant shown to be particularly beneficial in fighting prostate cancer. Grapefruit also contains limonoids: potent anti-carcinogens that may prevent cancerous cells from proliferating. Papaya is rich in papain, a digestive enzyme recognized for its anti-inflammatory properties.

Put the strawberries, raspberries and grapefruit through an electric juicer. Transfer to a blender or food processor and add the remaining ingredients. Blend until smooth. Serve the juice immediately.

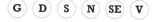

G D S N SE V

Nutritional information per serving
Kcals 102 | **Protein** 3.8g
Carbohydrates 31.9g, of which sugars 16.4g
Fat 0.4g, of which saturates 0.1g

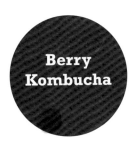

Berry Kombucha

1 small handful of blueberries
5 strawberries, stalks discarded
2 handfuls of red grapes
1 apple
60ml/2fl oz/¼ cup **KOMBUCHA** (page 22) or **WATER KEFIR** (page 22)
½ tsp **CAMU CAMU** powder, or **BAOBAB** powder or **ACAI BERRY** powder

Rich in anthocyanins and phenols, berries are nutrient-dense powerhouses and the perfect anti-ageing food. Red grapes supply the polyphenol resveratrol, which has been shown to help protect the body, and especially the skin, from free-radical damage. This is an excellent juice for reinvigorating your skin and boosting your immune health.

Put the blueberries, strawberries, grapes and apple through an electric juicer, then stir in the kombucha and the camu camu powder. Serve immediately.

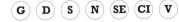

(G) (D) (S) (N) (SE) (CI) (V)

Nutritional information per serving
Kcals 165 | **Protein** 3.2g
Carbohydrates 60.3g, of which sugars 32.3g
Fat 0.3g, of which saturates 0g

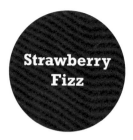

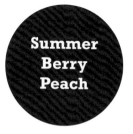

12 strawberries, stalks discarded
1 lime, peeled
2 apples
1 POMEGRANATE
60ml/2fl oz/¼ cup WATER KEFIR or
   COCONUT KEFIR (page 22), or fizzy
   water and ¼ tsp PROBIOTIC powder

A beautiful crimson juice, this
strawberry mix is light, refreshing and
ideal for boosting your digestive health
– especially because it also contains
gut-friendly kefir. If kefir is not available,
however, simply dilute the juice with
fizzy water with a little probiotic powder.

Put the strawberries, lime and apples
through an electric juicer. Cut the
pomegranate in half and squeeze the juice
into a bowl. Stir the pomegranate juice and
water kefir into the strawberry mixture.
Serve immediately.

(G) (D) (S) (N) (SE) (V)

Nutritional information per serving
Kcals 138 | **Protein** 2.2g
Carbohydrates 33.1g, of which sugars 31.6g
Fat 0.4g, of which saturates 0g

2 handfuls of raspberries
2 peaches, pitted
1 lime, peeled
1 apple
½ tsp CHIA SEEDS
½ tsp MAQUI BERRY powder or
   ACAI BERRY powder
5 COCONUT ICE CUBES (page 22) or
   ice cubes

This fruity cooler marries the wonderful
flavours of raspberries and peaches –
a winning combination for a cooling
summer drink. The chia seeds make
the juice slightly thicker and provide
essential omega-3 fats, together with
protein and calcium.

Put all the ingredients, except the chia
seeds, maqui berry powder and ice, through
an electric juicer. Transfer to a blender
or food processor and add the remaining
ingredients. Blend to create a slushy drink.
Serve immediately.

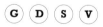

Nutritional information per serving
Kcals 129 | **Protein** 3.8g
Carbohydrates 24.3g, of which sugars 23.1g
Fat 1.9g, of which saturates 0.2g

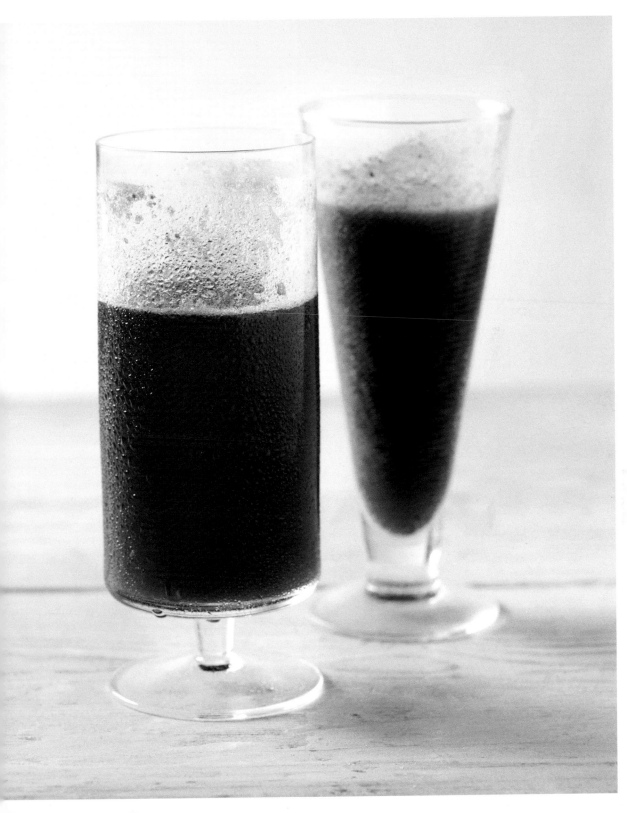

Acai Berry Refresher

¼ watermelon
100g/3½oz strawberries, stalks discarded
½ tsp ACAI BERRY powder
¼ tsp BAOBAB powder
1 tbsp DRIED MULBERRIES, or INCAN BERRIES or GOJI BERRIES
60ml/2fl oz/¼ cup KOMBUCHA (page 22)

This juice is a refreshing immune-boosting, gut-friendly drink. It is also well supplied with antioxidants, including the anti-ageing phenolic phytochemicals, anthocyanins and resveratrol. Blending in mulberries helps to thicken the juice, and the addition of baobab powder gives it a light, citrus tang.

Cut the watermelon flesh away from the peel. Discard the peel. Put the strawberries and watermelon through an electric juicer. Transfer to a blender or food processor and add the remaining ingredients, then blend until smooth. Serve immediately.

Health Benefits
Sweet-flavoured mulberries make an ideal snack to rejuvenate the body. Each berry is an encapsulation of nutrients, especially iron, calcium, vitamin C and plenty of anti-ageing antioxidants, including resveratrol. Adding a handful of mulberries to a smoothie provides additional fibre and protein.

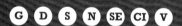

Nutritional information per serving
Kcals 158 | Protein 2.2g
Carbohydrates 35.1g, of which sugars 33g
Fat 2g, of which saturates 0.4g

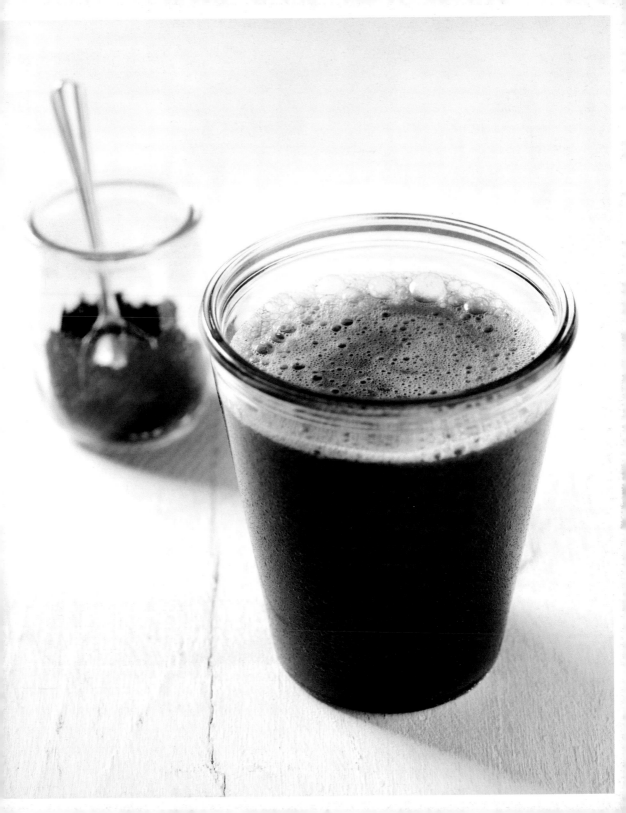

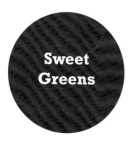

Sweet Greens

1 large handful of green grapes
1 pear
1 lime, peeled
1 handful of spinach
½ cucumber
¼ tsp **MATCHA GREEN TEA** powder

Light and refreshing, this green juice is hydrating, invigorating and loaded with antioxidants. Matcha contains 137 times the antioxidants of regular green tea. It is rich in the amino acid L-theanine and, together with a little caffeine, provides you with a sustained energy boost, creating a state of mental alertness and boosting concentration.

Put all the ingredients, except the matcha, through an electric juicer, then stir in the matcha. (Alternatively, transfer to a blender or food processor and process to blend in the matcha.) Serve immediately.

(G) (D) (S) (N) (SE) (V)

Nutritional information per serving
Kcals 165 | **Protein** 3.7g
Carbohydrates 38.3g, of which sugars 36.3g
Fat 0.7g, of which saturates 0.1g

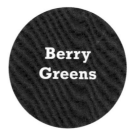

Berry Greens

1 handful of raspberries
1 handful of strawberries, stalks discarded
1 handful of spinach or watercress
1 apple
1 pear
¼ tsp **GREEN SUPERFOOD** powder, such as **WHEATGRASS**, **BARLEY GRASS** or **SPIRULINA** powder

If you're not usually enthusiastic about green juices, you may prefer this version based on berries – a reviving, power-packed juice containing antioxidants and energizing nutrients, including B vitamins, magnesium, potassium and iron. For a light-green juice, opt for wheatgrass or barley grass. If you like a darker, stronger protein-packed option, however, choose spirulina.

Put all the ingredients, except the green superfood powder, through an electric juicer, then stir in the superfood powder. Serve immediately.

 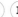

(G) (D) (S) (N) (SE) (CI) (V)

Nutritional information per serving
Kcals 119 | **Protein** 2.4g
Carbohydrates 27.9g, of which sugars 26.5g
Fat 0.5g, of which saturates 0g

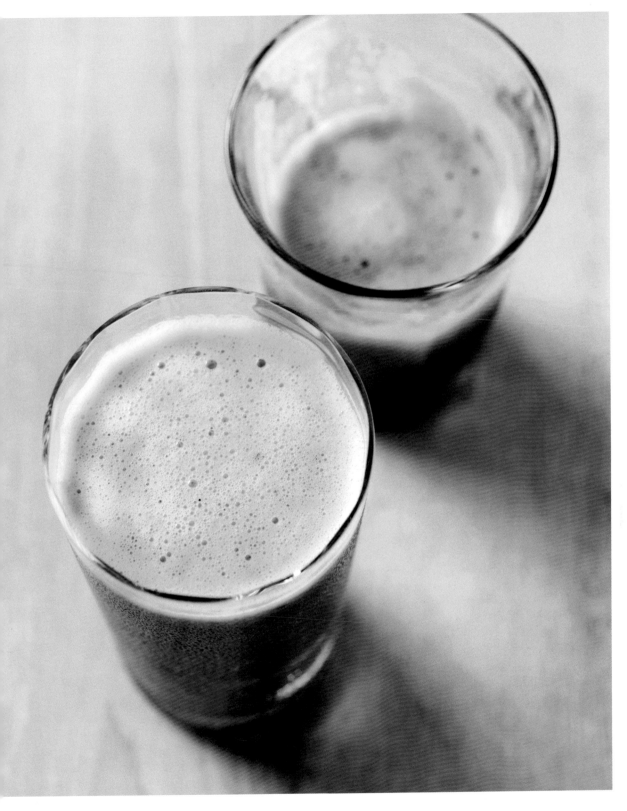

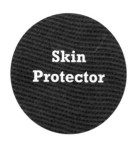

Skin Protector

½ cantaloupe melon
2 carrots
¼–½ tsp BAOBAB powder, to taste
1 tbsp GOJI BERRIES
1 tbsp COLLAGEN powder

If you're a sun worshipper and like to soak up the sun's rays, drink this juice for natural skin protection. Foods rich in carotenoids, such as melon and carrots, help to protect the skin against free-radical damage from sun exposure. They also contain lots of vitamin C, which has benefits for rejuvenating and repairing the skin, as well as enhancing collagen production. Because the body produces decreasing amounts of collagen as it ages, adding collagen powder to the juice can help to keep your skin supple and youthful.

Cut the melon flesh away from the peel. Discard the peel. Put the melon and carrots through an electric juicer. Transfer to a blender or food processor and add the remaining ingredients, then blend until smooth. Serve immediately.

(G) (D) (S) (N) (SE) (CI)

Nutritional information per serving
Kcals 182 | **Protein** 14.7g
Carbohydrates 29g, of which sugars 27.5g
Fat 1.3g, of which saturates 0.1g

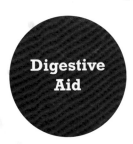

Digestive Aid

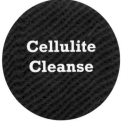

Cellulite Cleanse

½ small pineapple, skin cut off
1 apple
1cm/½in piece of root ginger, peeled
1 tsp organic apple cider vinegar
1 lemon, peeled
1 tbsp ALOE VERA juice

Alleviate indigestion by sipping
this invigorating juice. It's light and
refreshing and is ideal taken first thing
in the morning. The apple cider vinegar
will stimulate your digestive juices and
the ginger will ease feelings of nausea
while promoting digestion. Organic cider
vinegar is additive-free; the combination
of the vitamins it contains and its pH
level helps to detoxify the body, speed up
the metabolism and support digestion.

Put all the ingredients, except the aloe vera,
through an electric juicer, then stir in the
aloe vera. Serve immediately.

(G) (D) (S) (N) (SE) (V)

Nutritional information per serving
Kcals 139 | **Protein** 1.5g
Carbohydrates 33.9g, of which sugars 32.3g
Fat 0.7g, of which saturates 0g

1 pink grapefruit, peeled
2 celery sticks
1 apple
125ml/4fl oz/½ cup chilled NETTLE,
   DANDELION or GYNOSTEMMA TEA

Grapefruit is a natural cleansing fruit,
rich in bioflavonoids to help strengthen
capillaries and prevent cellulite. This is
a wonderfully hydrating and cleansing
drink to help flush out toxins from the
body, which can be associated with
cellulite. Any chilled herbal tea can
be used in this recipe, but to stimulate
cleansing, try a herbal combination of
dandelion, nettle or fennel. Alternatively,
choose gynostemma – an amazing
herb renowned for its anti-ageing and
rejuvenating effects. The juice is also
a useful stress tonic.

Put all the ingredients, except the tea,
through an electric juicer, then stir in the
tea. Serve immediately.

(G) (D) (S) (N) (SE) (V)

Nutritional information per serving
Kcals 84 | **Protein** 2g
Carbohydrates 19.3g, of which sugars 18.4g
Fat 0.3g, of which saturates 0g

Natural
Anti-
Inflammatory
Fighter

¼ pineapple, skin cut off
1cm/½in piece of root ginger, peeled
2 large handfuls of blackberries
1 apple
½ tsp AMLA BERRY powder
¼ tsp ground TURMERIC
½ tsp OMEGA OIL BLEND or FLAXSEED OIL
1 tsp COLOSTRUM powder or GLUTAMINE powder

A range of ingredients with natural anti-inflammatory properties, plus supercharged foods, form the cornerstone of this juice, which will help to dampen inflammation in the body and assist healing. I recommend you take this if you suffer with an inflammatory or autoimmune condition.

Put the pineapple, ginger, blackberries and apple through an electric juicer. Transfer to a blender or food processor and add the remaining ingredients, then blend briefly to combine. Serve immediately.

Health Benefits
Turmeric is an extraordinary, healing herb. Research has demonstrated its amazing ability to lower inflammation, boost detoxification and support liver function. The super-antioxidants contained in turmeric help the body to protect itself from damage and may also prevent cognitive decline.

Nutritional information per serving
Kcals 160 | **Protein** 3.2g
Carbohydrates 29.2g, of which sugars 28.8g
Fat 3.2g, of which saturates 0.2g

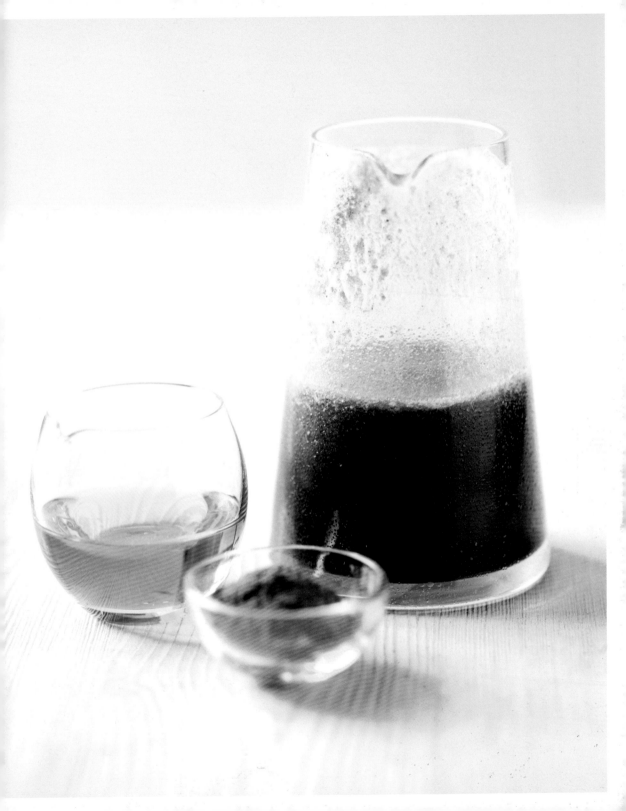

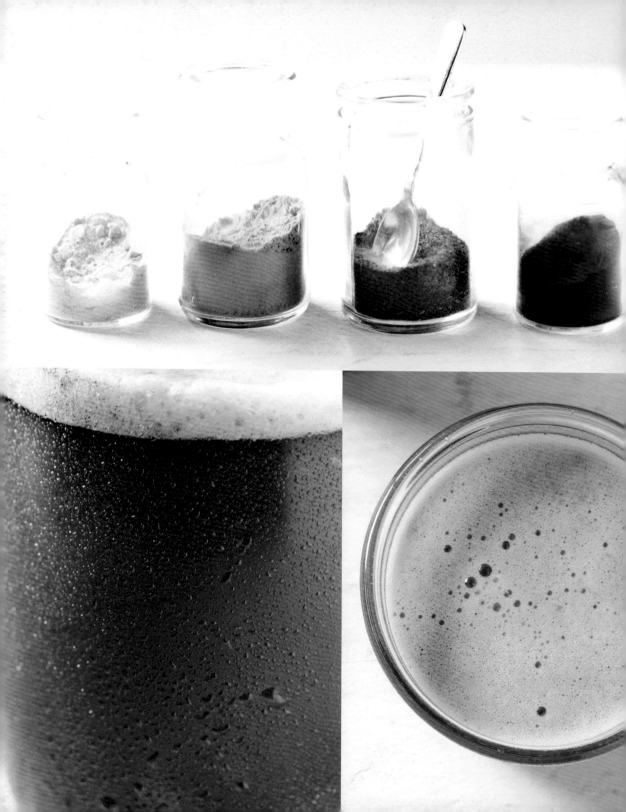

CHAPTER 2

VEGETABLE-BASED JUICES

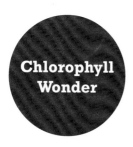

Chlorophyll Wonder

1 small handful of spinach leaves
1 small handful of kale leaves
1 pear
1 small lemon, peeled
½ small fennel bulb
½ cucumber
¼ tsp WHEATGRASS or BARLEY GRASS powder

Fabulously light, this green juice is crammed with nutrients to refresh and energize your body. Kale and spinach are excellent sources of minerals, including magnesium, iron, potassium and calcium. Adding a supergrass such as wheatgrass or barley grass provides concentrated nutrients and chlorophyll, making this an exceptionally alkalizing and cleansing juice.

Put all the ingredients, except the wheatgrass, through an electric juicer, then stir in the wheatgrass. Serve immediately.

  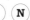

Nutritional information per serving
Kcals 86 | **Protein** 2.7g
Carbohydrates 17.9g, of which sugars 17.8g
Fat 0.8g, of which saturates 0.1g

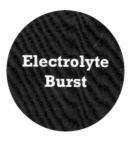

Electrolyte Burst

½ cucumber
1 celery stick
1 lime, peeled
1 apple
1 small handful of mint leaves
2 handfuls of spinach
60ml/2fl oz/¼ cup COCONUT WATER
3 ice cubes, to serve (optional)

This hydrating juice contains all the electrolytes our cells need to function at their best. Celery is rich in sodium and potassium, while cucumber, with its extremely high water content, is refreshing and cooling. Using coconut water gives the perfect balance of sodium, magnesium, potassium and calcium to energize the body rapidly.

Put all the ingredients, except the coconut water and ice, if using, through an electric juicer. Pour in the coconut water and serve over ice cubes, if you like.

 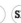

Nutritional information per serving
Kcals 60 | **Protein** 2.2g
Carbohydrates 11.4g, of which sugars 9.1g
Fat 0.6g, of which saturates 0g

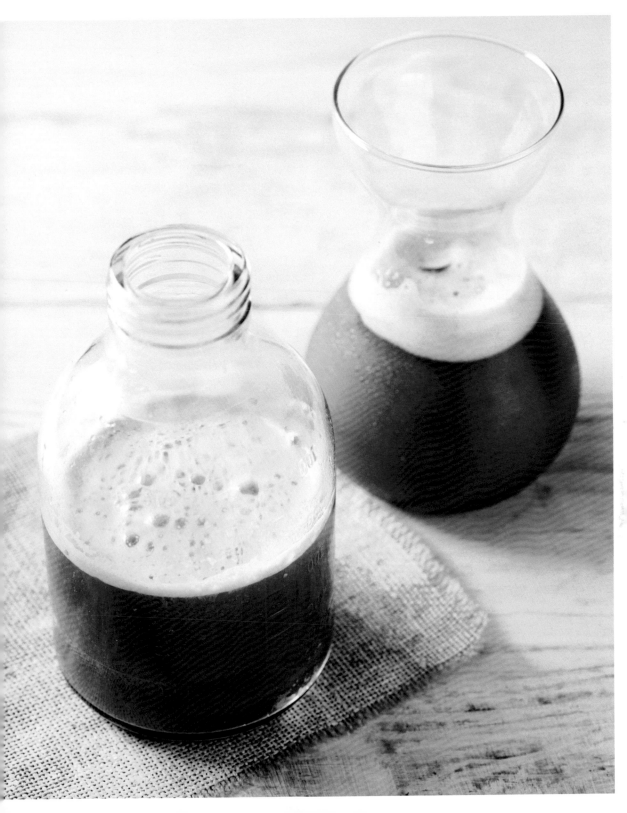

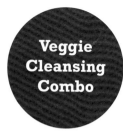

Veggie Cleansing Combo

2 carrots
1 apple
1 beetroot
½–1 lemon, to taste, peeled
¼ cucumber
1cm/½in piece of root ginger, peeled
5 drops of **MILK THISTLE** tincture

Beetroot, well known for its liver-cleansing properties, is a key ingredient in this revitalizing juice, which is enhanced further by the addition of milk thistle. Lemon, ginger, cucumber and apple balance the strong flavours of the root vegetables perfectly, giving the juice a pleasant savoury taste.

Put all the ingredients, except the milk thistle tincture, through an electric juicer, then stir in the milk thistle. Serve the juice immediately.

(G) (D) (S) (N) (SE) (V)

Nutritional information per serving
Kcals 73 | **Protein** 1.7g
Carbohydrates 15.6g, of which sugars 15.3g
Fat 0.4g, of which saturates 0.1g

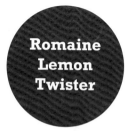

Romaine Lemon Twister

1 romaine or cos lettuce
1 handful of **ALFALFA SPROUTS**
1 large handful of green grapes
1 lemon, peeled
1 small pear
½ cucumber
¼ tsp MSM powder

Rich in vitamin C, romaine lettuce also contains vitamin K, which is essential for bone health. Alfalfa sprouts are also added to this juice to provide antioxidants, magnesium and calcium – important for healthy muscles and nerves. This is a wonderful juice to keep you looking radiant, containing silicon for healthy skin, hair and nails, and a beautifying boost from MSM powder.

Put all the ingredients, except the MSM powder, through an electric juicer, then stir in the MSM powder. Serve immediately.

(G) (D) (S) (N) (SE) (V)

Nutritional information per serving
Kcals 122 | **Protein** 2.3g
Carbohydrates 29.6g, of which sugars 29g
Fat 0.5g, of which saturates 0g

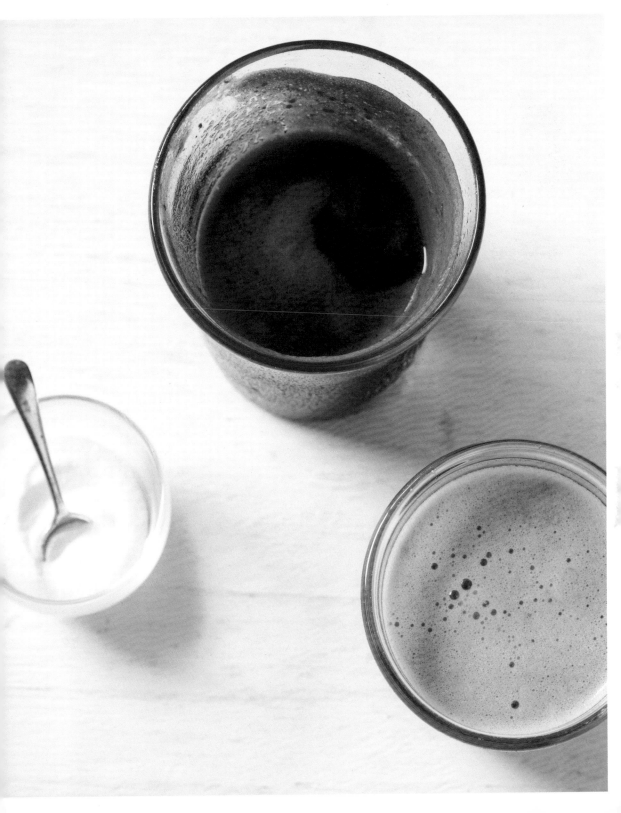

Lemon Green Cleanser

½–1 lemon, to taste, peeled
¼ pineapple, skin cut off
1 large handful of parsley leaves and stalks
1 apple
2 celery sticks
¼ cucumber
¼ tsp **CHLORELLA or SPIRULINA** powder
¼ tsp **WHEATGRASS** powder (optional)

Kick-start the day with this refreshing juice. The combination of tart lemon, parsley and supergreens makes this a perfect juice to hydrate and cleanse the body rapidly. Parsley contains folate and iron – essential to keep your energy levels high throughout the day. For an additional cleansing boost, add some wheatgrass powder.

Put all the ingredients, except the chlorella and wheatgrass powder, if using, through an electric juicer, then stir in the spirulina and wheatgrass powder. Serve immediately.

Health Benefits

Toxic build-up can lead to fatigue, aching joints, poor digestion and low mood, but one of the most effective nutritional strategies to fight this is to include green algae, such as chlorella, regularly in your diet. Prized for its natural detoxification abilities, chlorella can help bind to, and eliminate, heavy metals and certain chemicals, such as pesticides, from the body. The chlorophyll contained in chlorella rapidly oxygenates the body, enhancing your ability to focus and concentrate as well as strengthening your immune system.

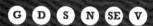

Nutritional information per serving
Kcals 85 | **Protein** 2.2g
Carbohydrates 17.2g, of which sugars 17g
Fat 0.6g, of which saturates 0g

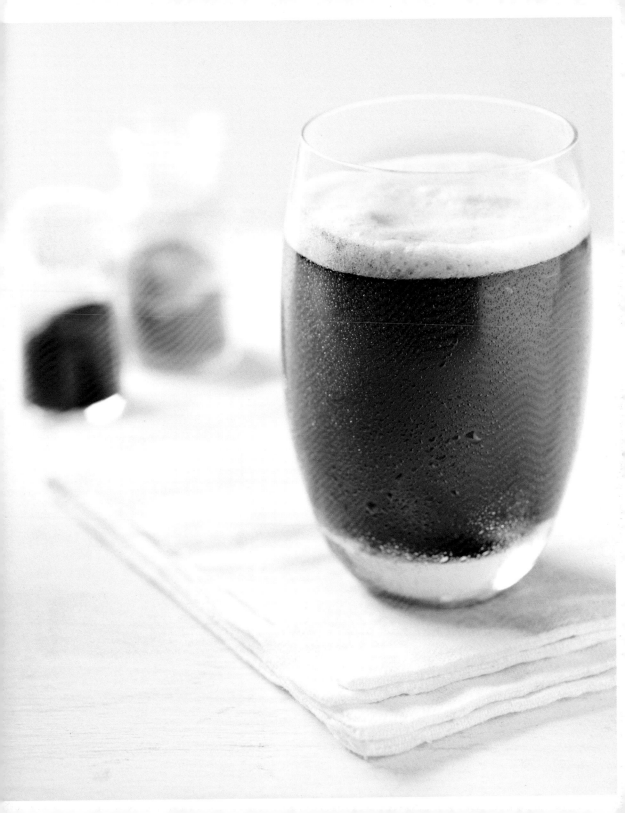

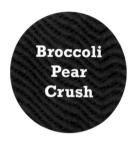

Broccoli Pear Crush

2 handfuls of broccoli
1 pear
½ lime, peeled
½ cucumber
¼ tsp **MORINGA LEAF** powder, **WHEATGRASS** powder or **GREEN SUPERFOOD BLEND**
8 **COCONUT ICE CUBES** (page 22) or ice cubes

With its refreshing tang, this green juice is packed with the health benefits of cruciferous vegetables. Broccoli is an amazing food. Rich in compounds known as glucosinolates to assist detoxification, broccoli helps to lower inflammation and prevent cancer, and moringa leaf powder boosts the body's immune system. Blend in the ice to create a slushy drink – just sip through a straw and savour!

Put all the ingredients, except the moringa powder and ice, through an electric juicer, then transfer to a blender or food processor and add the moringa powder and ice. Blend together until slushy. Serve immediately.

 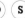

Nutritional information per serving
Kcals 96 | **Protein** 4.6g
Carbohydrates 16.5g, of which sugars 16.3g
Fat 1g, of which saturates 0.2g

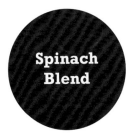

Spinach Blend

1 handful of spinach leaves
1 kiwi fruit, peeled
1 apple
1 handful of blueberries
½ cucumber
1 tsp **CHIA SEEDS**
⅛–¼ tsp **SPIRULINA** powder, to taste

Chia seeds plump up in the juice when soaked and blended, making this deep-green mix rich and thick. Chia seeds not only improve digestion but also help you to feel fuller for longer, making them excellent for weight loss.

Put all the ingredients, except the chia seeds and spirulina, through an electric juicer. Add the chia seeds and spirulina, and leave the juice to stand for 5 minutes. Transfer to a blender or food processor and blend until smooth. Serve immediately.

(**G**) (**D**) (**S**) (**N**) (**CI**) (**V**)

Nutritional information per serving
Kcals 95 | **Protein** 2.6g
Carbohydrates 17.6g, of which sugars 16.4g
Fat 1.5g, of which saturates 0.1g

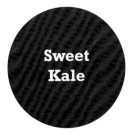

Sweet Kale

1 large handful of kale
1 peach or nectarine, pitted
1 apple
½ cucumber
¼ tsp **BAOBAB** powder or **CAMU CAMU** powder

Kale is an incredibly nourishing food, because it is abundant in vitamins K, C, A and B as well as minerals such as calcium, magnesium and iron. Known for its anti-cancer properties, kale contains many anti-inflammatory nutrients, including omega-3 fats. The addition of baobab powder gives this juice a slightly citrus tang as well as a massive boost of vitamin C.

Put all the ingredients, except the baobab powder, through an electric juicer, then stir in the baobab powder. (Alternatively, transfer to a blender or food processor and process to blend in the powder.) Serve the juice immediately.

(**G**) (**D**) (**S**) (**N**) (**SE**) (**CI**) (**V**)

Nutritional information per serving
Kcals 80 | **Protein** 2.8g
Carbohydrates 27.7g, of which sugars 13.6g
Fat 0.4g, of which saturates 0g

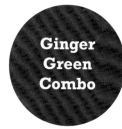

Ginger Green Combo

Pictured>

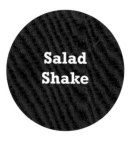

Salad Shake

2 green apples
1 small courgette
½ cucumber
½ romaine or cos lettuce
1 small lemon, peeled
1cm/½in piece of root ginger, peeled
¼ tsp MORINGA LEAF powder (optional)

The volatile oils present in fresh ginger are beautifully soothing to the digestive system, as well as easing nausea and stomach upsets. This light-green juice is high in vitamin C and beta-carotene, which help to prevent the oxidation of cholesterol. Romaine lettuce is a good source of B vitamins, including folate, to support cardiovascular health as well as promoting energy levels. You can supercharge this juice by adding a little moringa leaf powder.

Put all the ingredients, except the moringa powder, if using, through an electric juicer, then stir in the moringa powder. Serve the juice immediately.

G D S N SE V

Nutritional information per serving
Kcals 94 | **Protein** 2.8g
Carbohydrates 18.3g, of which sugars 18g
Fat 0.7g, of which saturates 0.1g

2 large tomatoes
2 small celery sticks
¼ cucumber
½ red pepper, deseeded
1 small handful of parsley leaves
  and stalks
2 tsp nutritional yeast flakes
1¼ tsp MEDICINAL MUSHROOM
  powder, or CHAGA or MACA powder
¼ tsp SEAWEED GRANULES or
  NORI SHEET, crumbled
Himalayan sea salt or sea salt, to taste
  (optional)

Enjoy the savoury flavour of a fresh salad in a glass. Invigorating and hydrating, this juice combines the saltiness of celery with the sweetness of tomatoes and red pepper.

Put all the ingredients, except the yeast flakes, mushroom powder, seaweed and salt, if using, through an electric juicer. Transfer to a blender or food processor and add the remaining ingredients. Blend until smooth.

 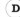 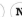
G D S N SE CI V

Nutritional information per serving
Kcals 74 | **Protein** 5.3g
Carbohydrates 10.6g, of which sugars 8.4g
Fat 1.1g, of which saturates 0.2g

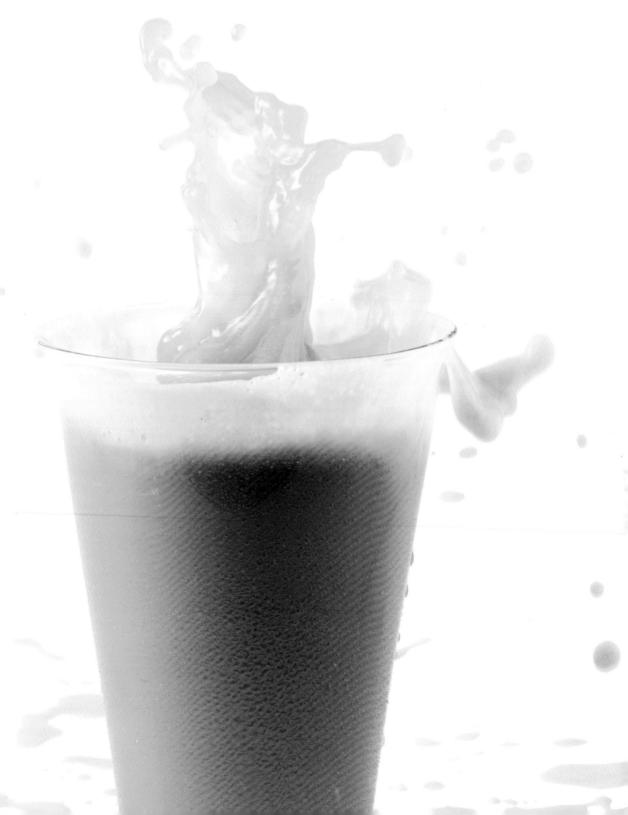

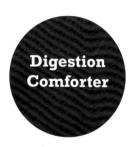

Digestion Comforter

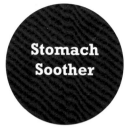

Stomach Soother

½ small fennel bulb
1 small handful of ALFALFA SPROUTS
5 mint leaves
1 apple
1 lime, peeled
½ cucumber
¼ tsp PROBIOTIC powder

100g/3½oz green cabbage
1 pear
1 apple
1 celery stick
½ cucumber
¼ tsp CAMU CAMU powder, or BAOBAB powder or ACAI BERRY powder
¼ tsp PROBIOTIC powder

When your digestive system needs a little support, reach for this soothing green juice. Fennel contains anethole, a volatile oil that stimulates secretion of the digestive and gastric juices, thereby reducing inflammation of the stomach and intestines, and aiding digestion. Mint provides a refreshing zing to this juice and calms muscle spasms, relieving flatulence and reducing abdominal cramps.

Cabbage juice is known for its ability to heal stomach ulcers and soothe the digestive tract, probably due to a range of digestion-friendly compounds that it contains, including glucosinolates, polyphenols and the amino acid-like substance called glutamine. The addition of probiotic powder further supports digestive health, and the camu camu powder adds a tangy, vitamin-C boost.

Put all the ingredients through an electric juicer. Serve immediately.

Put all the ingredients, except the camu camu powder and probiotic powder, through an electric juicer. Stir in the camu camu powder and probiotic powder, and serve immediately.

(G) (S) (N) (SE)

(G) (S) (N) (SE) (CI)

Nutritional information per serving
Kcals 50 | **Protein** 1.7g
Carbohydrates 9.5g, of which sugars 9.4g
Fat 0.4g, of which saturates 0g

Nutritional information per serving
Kcals 106 | **Protein** 3.7g
Carbohydrates 32.7g, of which sugars 18.6g
Fat 0.7g, of which saturates 0.1g

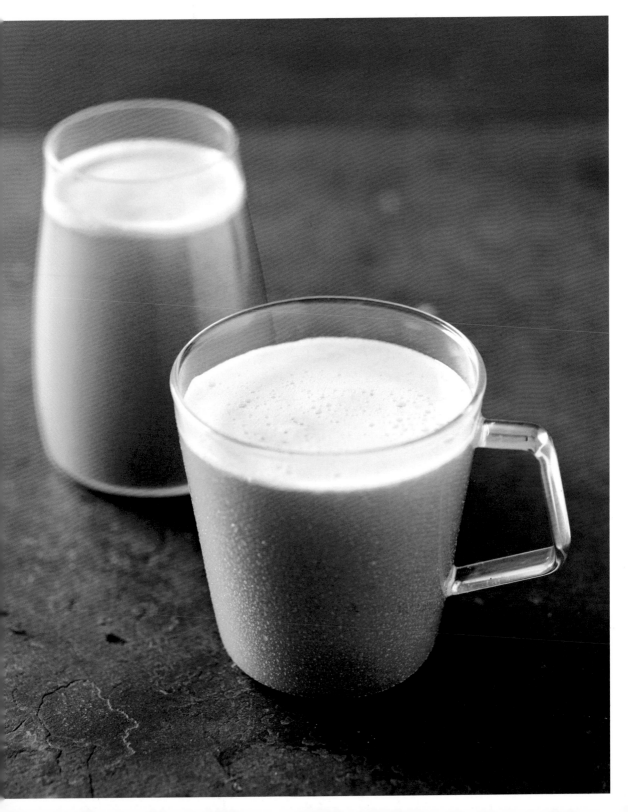

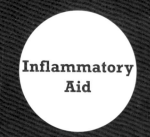

Inflammatory Aid

2 **carrots**
¼ **pineapple, skin cut off**
½ **lemon, peeled**
1cm/½in **piece of root ginger, peeled (optional)**
¼ **ripe mango, chopped**
¼ **tsp ground TURMERIC**
½ **tsp FLAXSEED OIL**
¼ **tsp BEE POLLEN or HONEY, plus a little extra, to serve**

This vibrant orange juice is bursting with anti-inflammatory nutrients. Pineapple is rich in bromelain, a digestive enzyme shown to help reduce inflammation, while the addition of turmeric provides plenty of curcumin – the active ingredient known for its anti-inflammatory properties. A dash of omega-rich flaxseed oil and bee pollen boosts the healing benefits of this juice further.

Put the carrots, pineapple, lemon and ginger, if using, through an electric juicer. Transfer to a blender or food processor and add the remaining ingredients, then process until smooth. Pour into glasses and sprinkle over a little bee pollen to serve.

Health Benefits

Bee pollen has been used for centuries. People from many different cultures have also taken it as a natural tonic to boost the body's energy and immune systems. It contains 40 per cent protein and all the essential amino acids, enzymes, fats and various vitamins, minerals and antioxidants to help regulate the immune system. Bee pollen stimulates an increase in physical and mental abilities, especially concentration and memory. It activates sluggish metabolic functions and strengthens the cardiovascular and respiratory systems. Because it has an exceptionally high antioxidant activity, it helps to protect the liver and balances the hormones. It also greatly increases energy levels, making it a favourite among athletes.

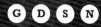

Nutritional information per serving
Kcals 97 | **Protein** 1.4g
Carbohydrates 18.1g, of which sugars 17.6g
Fat 2g, of which saturates 0.3g

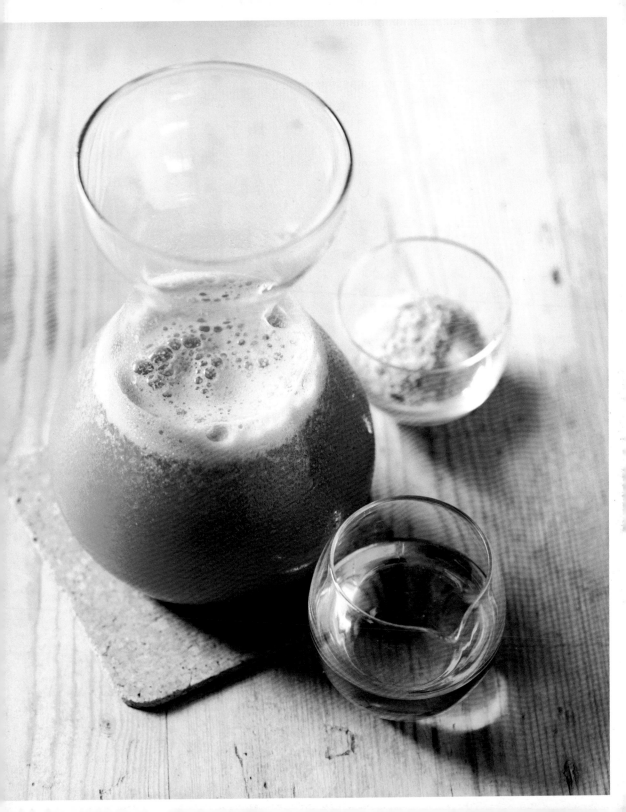

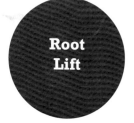

Root Lift

Pictured>

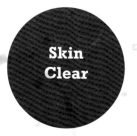

Skin Clear

1 parsnip
2 carrots
¼ celeriac, peeled
2 apples
1 tsp MSM powder or flakes

Give your hair and skin an inner makeover with this tasty, savoury juice. Parsnips create a creamy texture to the juice as well as being rich in folate. The celeriac and carrots are good sources of phytonutrients, B vitamins and minerals, including iron, phosphorus and calcium. Methylsulfonylmethane (MSM) powder is an organic sulphur compound that can be found naturally in a number of foods, and in small amounts it is also produced in the human body; sulphur is essential for the formation of collagen and keratin, essential for healthy hair, skin and nails.

Put all the ingredients, except the MSM powder, through an electric juicer, then stir in the MSM powder. Serve immediately.

Nutritional information per serving
Kcals 127 | **Protein** 4.4g
Carbohydrates 28g, of which sugars 22.9g
Fat 1.1g, of which saturates 0.2g

1 handful of kale
1 celery stick
¼ cucumber
1 orange, peeled
¼ pineapple, skin cut off
¼ avocado, peeled
1–2 tsp ALOE VERA juice, to taste
60ml/2fl oz/¼ cup cold GREEN TEA

Beautiful skin starts from within. Promote clear skin with the antioxidant-rich ingredients in this juice: aloe vera juice has been used for thousands of years internally and externally as a skin healer; avocado contains healthy fats to nourish and repair skin cells and calm inflammation; and green tea is loaded with antioxidants to protect the skin.

Put all the ingredients, except the avocado, aloe vera and tea, through an electric juicer. Transfer to a blender or food processor and add the remaining ingredients, then blend until smooth. Serve immediately.

 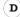 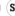 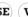

Nutritional information per serving
Kcals 135 | **Protein** 3g
Carbohydrates 18.5g, of which sugars 18.4g
Fat 5.5g, of which saturates 1.1g

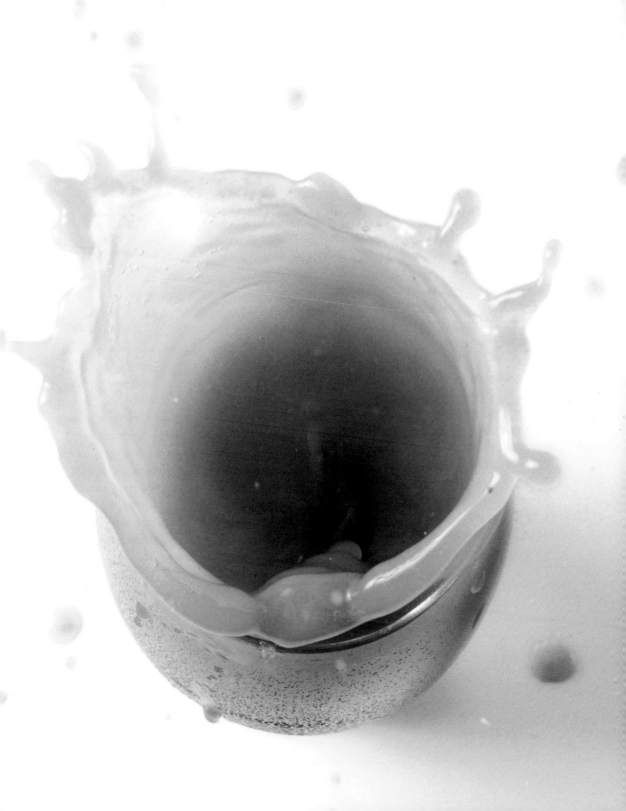

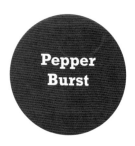

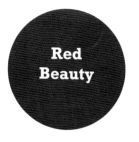

Pepper Burst

1 red pepper, deseeded
½ orange pepper, deseeded
2 large carrots
½–1 lemon, to taste, peeled
⅓ cucumber
1 tsp COLLAGEN powder
½ tsp FLAXSEED OIL or OMEGA OIL
   BLEND (optional)

You could call this Botox in a juice!
It's a light, savoury juice that is the
perfect antidote to tired and dull-looking
skin. The nourishing and revitalizing
qualities are the carotenoids, vitamin C
and sulphur contained in the peppers.
Collagen powder is added to keep the
skin glowing, but it can also help to
soothe sore joints. For additional benefit
to the skin, you could stir in a little
flaxseed oil too.

Put all the ingredients, except the collagen
powder and flaxseed oil, if using, through
an electric juicer, then stir in the collagen
powder and oil. Serve immediately.

   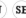 G D S N SE

Nutritional information per serving
Kcals 94 | **Protein** 5g
Carbohydrates 12.2g, of which sugars 11.8g
Fat 2.6g, of which saturates 0.4g

Red Beauty

4 small tomatoes
½ cucumber
1 apple
1 carrot
1 tsp FLAXSEED OIL
1 tbsp ALOE VERA juice

For glowing, vibrant skin, savour this
delicious antioxidant-packed juice.
Tomatoes are replete with the anti-ageing
nutrient lycopene as well as vitamin
C, and carrots provide plenty of beta-
carotene. All of these are important
nutrients for protecting the skin from
damage as well as encouraging cell
repair and healing. Because the juice also
contains aloe vera, it's ideal for tackling
scars and blemishes, and the potassium
in tomatoes makes it wonderfully
hydrating and cleansing.

Put all the ingredients, except the flaxseed
oil and aloe vera, through an electric juicer,
then stir in the flaxseed oil and aloe vera.
Serve immediately.

   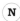 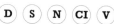 G D S N CI V

Nutritional information per serving
Kcals 129 | **Protein** 2.7g
Carbohydrates 18.3g, of which sugars 18.1g
Fat 4.7g, of which saturates 0.6g

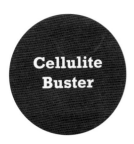

Cellulite Buster

2 celery sticks
1 handful of parsley leaves and stalks
1 cucumber
¼ pineapple, skin cut off
1 lemon, peeled
2 tsp LECITHIN granules

If you're looking for a natural way to smooth the orange peel-like skin indicative of cellulite, then sip this juice. The light and cleansing ingredients will help to remove toxins and waste materials from your body. Lecithin granules are rich in phospholipids, essential for all cells, and they also help to emulsify fat and excrete it from the body, so they are ideal for promoting weight loss.

Put all the ingredients, except the lecithin granules, through an electric juicer, then stir in the lecithin granules. (Alternatively, transfer to a blender or food processor and process to blend in the lecithin.) Serve immediately.

(G) (D) (N) (V)

Nutritional information per serving
Kcals 80 | **Protein** 1.9g
Carbohydrates 11.4g, of which sugars 11.3g
Fat 0.6g, of which saturates 0g

Iron Fortifier

1 large handful of watercress leaves
1 handful of parsley leaves and stalks
1 green apple
1 celery stick
½–1 lime, to taste, peeled
1 kiwi fruit, peeled
¼ tsp **PANAX GINSENG** tincture or ⅛ tsp **PANAX GINSENG** powder
⅛–¼ tsp **CHLORELLA** or **SPIRULINA** powder, to taste

If you're looking for a healthy pick-me-up for flagging energy levels, try this invigorating iron-rich juice. Both watercress and parsley provide iron and B vitamins, such as folate and B12, which the body needs for healthy red blood cells, and for mental and physical health.

Put all the ingredients, except the panax ginseng and chlorella, through an electric juicer. Stir in the panax ginseng and chlorella, and serve immediately.

Health Benefits
Panax ginseng has traditionally been used for its energy-giving properties to combat stress and improve mood. Various research studies have shown that it can improve cognitive function and memory, as well as stabilizing blood sugar levels, boosting circulation and reducing fatigue.

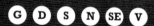

Nutritional information per serving
Kcals 70 | **Protein** 1.9g
Carbohydrates 14.9g, of which sugars 14.7g
Fat 0.7g, of which saturates 0.1g

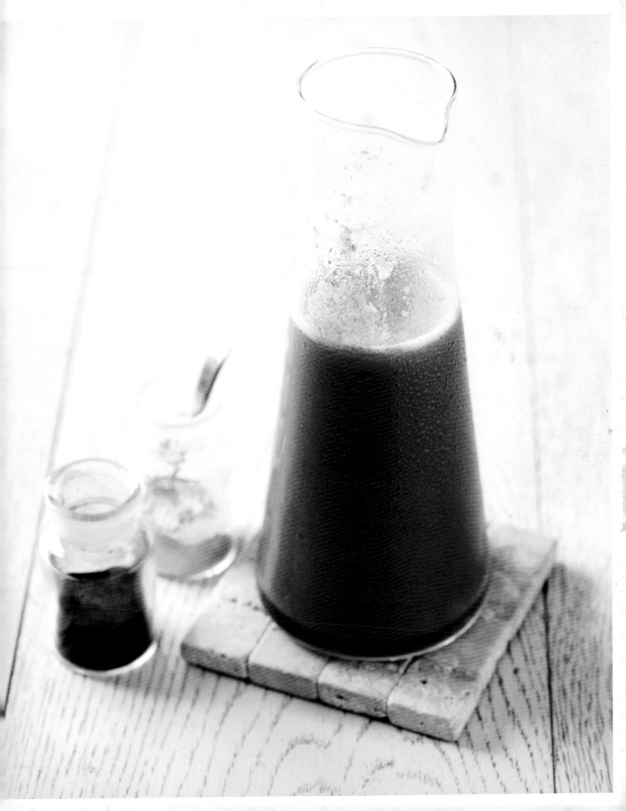

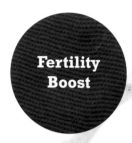

Fertility Boost

4 asparagus spears
1 handful of parsley leaves and stalks
2 celery sticks
½ cucumber
2 small apples
2 lemons, peeled
¼ tsp **SHATAVARI** powder or **MACA** powder

Shatavari is added to this juice for its ability to bring hormonal balance to women of all ages through the phytoestrogens it contains. Known to boost fertility, shatavari also relieves menopausal symptoms. Asparagus provides B vitamins, including folate, which are important for a healthy pregnancy, energy and lowering homocysteine, a compound produced by the body which, in excess, can affect fertility levels and increase the risk of cardiovascular disease and cognitive decline. In all, this is a wonderful tonic to nourish the whole body.

Put all the ingredients, except the shatavari powder, through an electric juicer. Transfer to a blender or food processor and add the shatavari powder, then blend until smooth. Serve the juice immediately.

(G) (D) (S) (N) (SE) (V)

Nutritional information per serving
Kcals 103 | **Protein** 4.2g
Carbohydrates 20.3g, of which sugars 20.1g
Fat 1g, of which saturates 0.1g

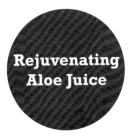

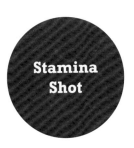

Stamina Shot

½ cantaloupe melon
1 handful of spinach leaves
1 handful of parsley leaves and stalks
1 lime, peeled
¼ cucumber
¼ tsp GINSENG powder or GINSENG tincture, or RHODIOLA

Need a quick energy burst? Try this stimulating green juice. Rich in iron and B vitamins, it will help to boost your energy levels. If you're feeling stressed, give this juice additional oomph with a little ginseng or rhodiola tincture.

Cut the melon flesh away from the peel. Discard the peel. Put all the ingredients, except the ginseng, through an electric juicer, then stir in the ginseng. Serve the juice immediately.

(G) (D) (S) (N) (SE) (V)

Nutritional information per serving
Kcals 68 | **Protein** 2.8g
Carbohydrates 13.6g, of which sugars 13.5g
Fat 0.6g, of which saturates 0g

Rejuvenating Aloe Juice

2 large handfuls of spinach leaves
¼ pineapple, skin cut off
1 lime, peeled
1 handful of mint leaves
2 celery sticks
1 tbsp ALOE VERA juice

Sip on this revitalizing tonic if you're feeling a little below par. It's refreshing and is designed to settle the digestive tract, calm inflammation and rejuvenate the body. Known as 'the plant of immortality' by the Egyptians, aloe is a mineral-rich supercharged food, which is beneficial for the whole digestive system, reducing Candida and promoting friendly bacteria. It also encourages healing and cell regeneration, and its anti-inflammatory properties make it effective for combating disorders such as indigestion, ulcers and heartburn.

Put all the ingredients, except the aloe vera, through an electric juicer, then stir in the aloe vera. Serve immediately.

(G) (D) (S) (N) (SE) (V)

Nutritional information per serving
Kcals 80 | **Protein** 2.1g
Carbohydrates 16.4g, of which sugars 15.6g
Fat 0.8g, of which saturates 0.1g

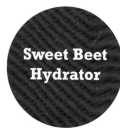

Sweet Beet Hydrator   *Pictured>*

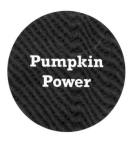

Pumpkin Power

1 beetroot
2 carrots
230g/8oz strawberries, stalks discarded
1 apple
125ml/4fl oz/½ cup COCONUT WATER

This ruby-pink juice is sweet and
light with ingredients that are superb
for rejuvenating and energizing the
body before a workout. Beetroot is a
unique source of phytonutrients, called
betalains, which have been shown to
provide antioxidant, anti-inflammatory
and detoxification qualities for the body.

Put all the ingredients, except the coconut
water, through an electric juicer, then stir
in the coconut water. Serve immediately.

(G) (D) (S) (SE) (CI) (V)

Nutritional information per serving
Kcals 153 | **Protein** 4g
Carbohydrates 32.1g, of which sugars 27.6g
Fat 0.8g, of which saturates 0.1g

250g/9oz pumpkin, peeled and cut
   into chunks
1 carrot
2 apples
1cm/½in piece of root ginger, peeled
½ tsp MACA powder
¼ tsp ground cinnamon, or to taste

Golden and creamy, this juice is
bursting with antioxidants – including
carotenoids and vitamin C, B vitamins,
manganese and magnesium – all of
which are important nutrients for energy
production. It's a wonderfully anti-
inflammatory juice, naturally sweet for
an energy lift and perfect for nourishing
the adrenal glands and immune system.

Put all the ingredients, except the maca
powder and cinnamon, through an electric
juicer, then stir in the maca and cinnamon.
Serve immediately.

(G) (D) (S) (N) (SE) (CI) (V)

Nutritional information per serving
Kcals 110 | **Protein** 2.7g
Carbohydrates 22.7g, of which sugars 21.3g
Fat 0.8g, of which saturates 0.3g

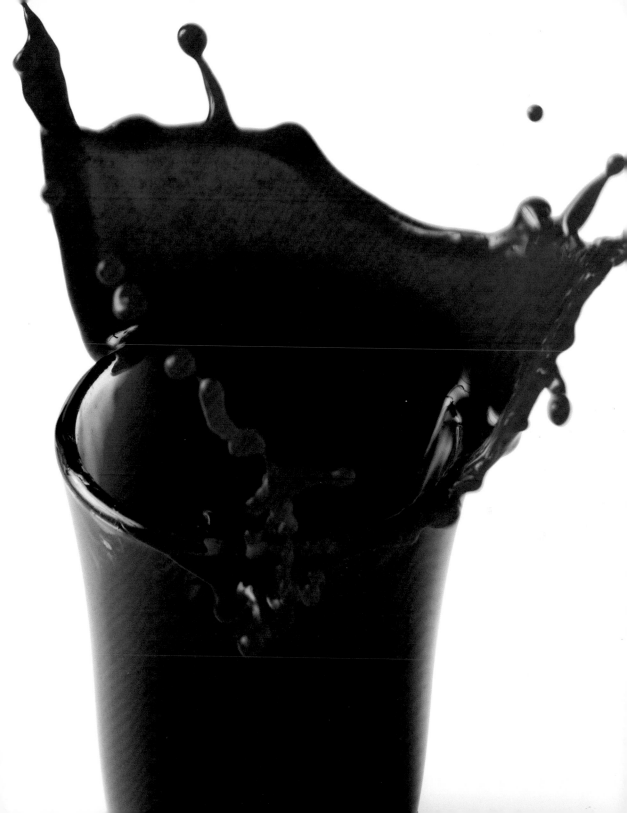

Beet and Berry Performance

1 beetroot
100g/3½oz/⅔ cup blueberries
120g/4¼oz/⅔ cup pitted fresh or frozen cherries
2 pears
1 lemon, peeled
a few drops of GINSENG tincture or ¼ tsp GINSENG powder
½ tsp ACAI BERRY powder
1 tbsp GLUTAMINE powder

Rich in nitrates, beetroot juice can help increase oxygenation throughout the body and, for this reason, it is a well-known sports-performance aid. The addition of antioxidant-rich fruits and glutamine powder makes this an excellent juice to aid recovery after exercise and for re-energizing the body.

Put all the ingredients, except the ginseng, acai berry powder and glutamine powder, through an electric juicer, then stir in the remaining ingredients. Serve immediately.

Health Benefits
Berries and cherries, and especially acai, are supercharged foods for athletes, because they contain high levels of flavonoids and anthocyanins, which are known for their antioxidant and anti-inflammatory benefits. Including juices, such as this one, regularly in the diet can help lower inflammation and improve recovery, allowing athletes to train harder for longer periods.

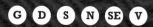

Nutritional information per serving
Kcals 281 | **Protein** 13.1g
Carbohydrates 60.7g, of which sugars 51.6g
Fat 1.5g, of which saturates 0g

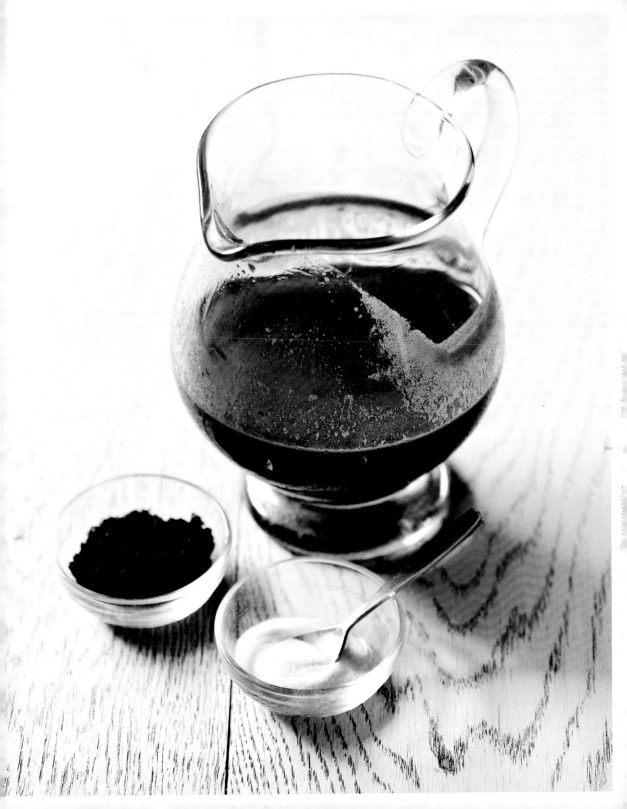

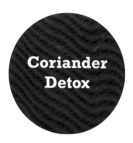

Coriander Detox

1 handful of coriander leaves and stalks
4 celery sticks
1 lime, peeled
1 handful of parsley leaves and stalks
2 apples
¼ tsp CHLORELLA powder or a few drops of CHLOROPHYLL liquid

Fresh coriander is a nutrient-dense herb containing volatile oils with beneficial phytonutrients. It is traditionally used to help the body detoxify heavy metals and toxins. This juice is further supercharged by stirring in a little chlorella or chlorophyll liquid. It's particularly useful to take as a New Year cleanse after the excesses of the festive season.

Put all the ingredients, except the chlorella, through an electric juicer, then stir in the chlorella. Serve immediately.

  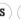

Nutritional information per serving
Kcals 47 | **Protein** 1.8g
Carbohydrates 9.5g, of which sugars 9.4g
Fat 0.5g, of which saturates 0g

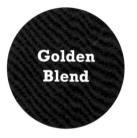

Golden Blend

3 large carrots
1 lemon, peeled
¼ cucumber
½ pear
1 apple
½ tsp FLAXSEED OIL or OMEGA OIL BLEND

This vibrant, zingy juice is packed with antioxidants, particularly carotenoids, which are known for their cancer-protective properties. Beta-carotene from the carrots is converted into vitamin A – an important vitamin for the eyes and skin, and for maintaining immune health. Omega-3 fats from the flaxseed oil give this juice an anti-inflammatory boost.

Put all the ingredients, except the flaxseed oil, through an electric juicer, then stir in the flaxseed oil. Serve immediately.

 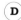

Nutritional information per serving
Kcals 118 | **Protein** 1.5g
Carbohydrates 22g, of which sugars 22g
Fat 2.4g, of which saturates 0.3g

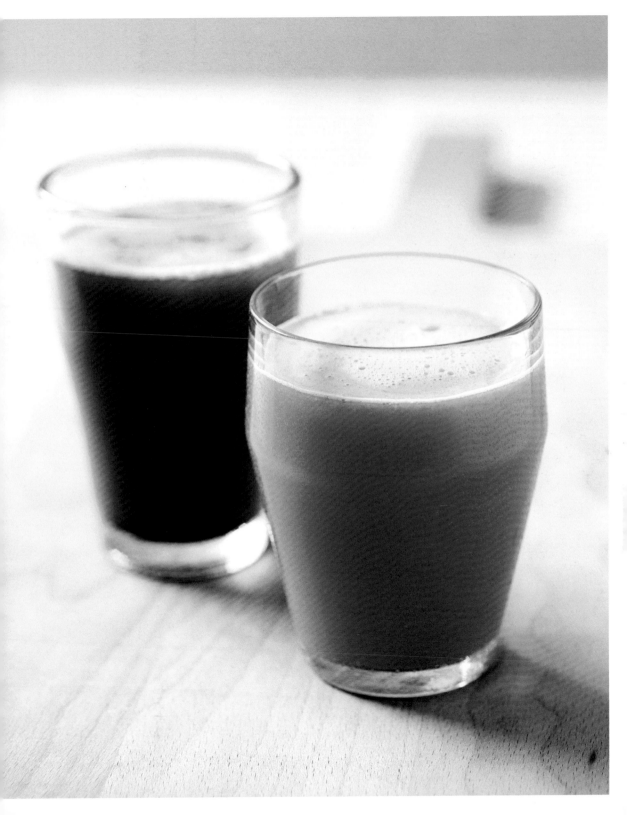

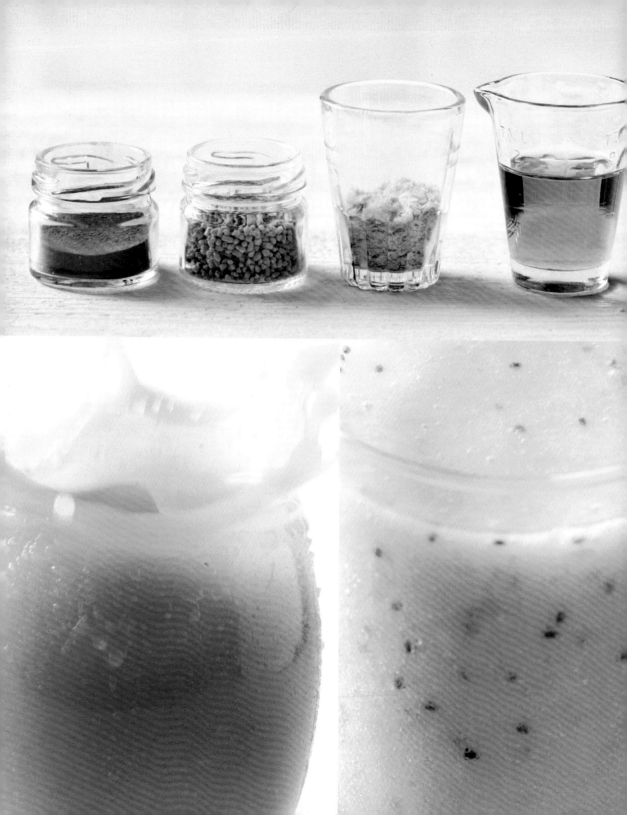

CHAPTER 3

ULTIMATE SMOOTHIES

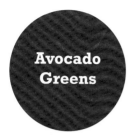

Avocado Greens

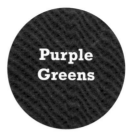

Purple Greens

¼ avocado, peeled
1 tsp COCONUT OIL
100g/3½oz fresh or frozen pineapple, chopped
juice of ½ lime
¼ tsp MORINGA LEAF powder, CHLORELLA or SPIRULINA powder
1 tsp ALOE VERA juice
2 tsp GLUTAMINE powder
½ tsp PROBIOTIC powder
200ml/7fl oz/scant 1 cup COCONUT WATER or water

Creamy avocado combines with coconut oil to create a velvety texture. This smoothie is particularly useful for soothing the digestive tract. It contains digestive enzymes from the pineapple, plus glutamine and probiotics to heal the gut, and aloe vera and moringa leaf powder for reducing inflammation.

Put all the ingredients into a blender or food processor and blend until smooth and creamy. Serve immediately.

 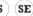 (SE)

Nutritional information per serving
Kcals 188 | **Protein** 9.2g
Carbohydrates 24g, of which sugars 10g
Fat 8.5g, of which saturates 3.6g

1 large handful of red grapes
1 large handful of frozen blueberries or mixed berries
2 pitted soft dried dates
½ tsp PURPLE CORN powder
½ tsp AMLA BERRY powder or ACAI BERRY powder
½ tsp vanilla extract
35g/1¼oz red cabbage, shredded
1 handful of purple kale, chopped

Purple kale and red cabbage are rich in anthocyanins, a phytonutrient with disease-fighting benefits. Purple corn has exceptional antioxidant properties to counter free-radical damage and promote cell health.

Put the grapes into a freezer bag. Exclude all the air, then seal and freeze overnight or until solid. Put the grapes and the remaining ingredients into a blender or food processor and blend until smooth and creamy. Add up to 100ml/3½ fl oz/generous ⅓ cup water to thin as needed. Serve immediately.

 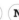 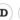

Nutritional information per serving
Kcals 150 | **Protein** 2.5g
Carbohydrates 32g, of which sugars 27.2g
Fat 1.3g, of which saturates 0g

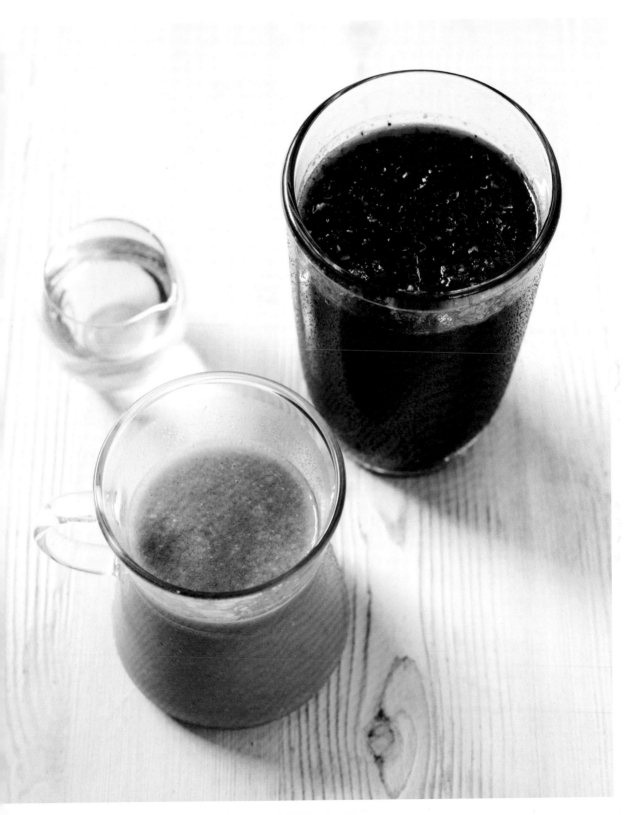

Brain Booster

1 small handful of blueberries, fresh or frozen
3 strawberries, stalks discarded, chopped
2 tsp SHELLED HEMP SEEDS
1 tsp ACAI BERRY powder
1 tbsp GOJI BERRIES
¼ tsp GINKGO powder or 2 drops of GINKGO tincture
½ tsp FLAXSEED OIL
½ tsp COCONUT OIL
¼ ripe avocado, peeled and chopped
100ml/3½fl oz/generous ⅓ cup POMEGRANATE juice, COCONUT WATER,
    cold GINKGO TEA or GREEN TEA

This smoothie has it all: healthy fats, protein and antioxidants to nourish and protect the brain. It's also rich and satisfying, thanks to the addition of avocado. If you're wanting an alternative to pomegranate juice and you can't find ginkgo powder or tincture, use matcha green tea powder or ginkgo tea instead.

Put all the ingredients into a blender or food processor and blend until smooth and creamy. Serve immediately.

Health Benefits
Ginkgo biloba is a Chinese herb from the leaves of the tree of the same name, and has been shown through centuries of use and research to be a powerful antioxidant. Rich in phytonutrients, including proanthocyanidins and flavonoids, it has been shown to protect the cells from oxidative damage. Ginkgo is particularly known for its ability to stimulate circulation, boost cognitive function and prevent memory loss.

    (G) (D) (S) (CI) (V)

Nutritional information per serving
Kcals 268 | **Protein** 4.1g
Carbohydrates 32g, of which sugars 29.1g
Fat 13.5g, of which saturates 2.7g

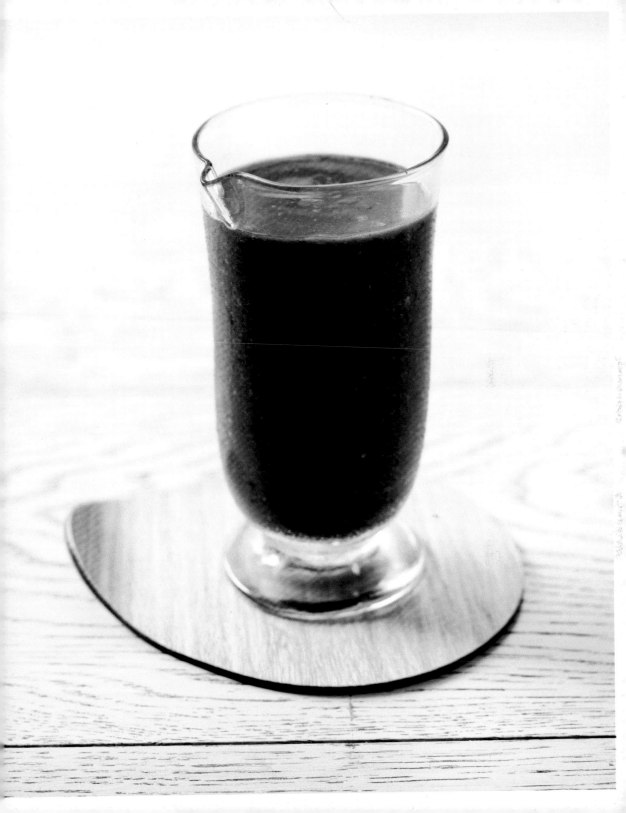

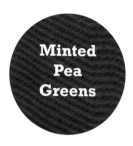

**Minted
Pea
Greens**

2 tsp COCONUT OIL, melted
1 tbsp unsweetened coconut flakes or desiccated coconut
1 tbsp chopped mint leaves
¼ tsp CAMU CAMU powder, or BAOBAB powder or ACAI BERRY powder
35g/1¼oz/¼ cup frozen or fresh raw, podded peas
¼ cucumber, chopped
¼ avocado, peeled and chopped
200ml/7fl oz/scant 1 cup COCONUT WATER
1 tbsp RAW CACAO NIBS
8 ice cubes or COCONUT ICE CUBES (page 22)
stevia, coconut sugar or xylitol (optional), to taste

This cooling and refreshing green smoothie has a little crunch from the cacao nibs. Because it can be made with frozen peas, you can enjoy summer freshness all year round, and your skin can benefit from the drink's hydrating properties. Camu camu powder or baobab adds a burst of nourishing vitamin C as well.

Put all the ingredients, except half the cacao nibs, the ice and stevia, if using, into a blender or food processor and blend until smooth and creamy. Add the ice and reserved cacao nibs and blend once more to retain some texture. Sweeten to taste if needed. Serve immediately.

(G) (D) (S) (SE) (CI) (V)

Nutritional information per serving
Kcals 340 | **Protein** 9g
Carbohydrates 45.9g, of which sugars 2.1g
Fat 25.5g, of which saturates 16.4g

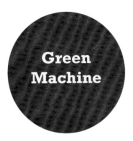

Green Machine

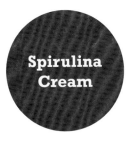

Spirulina Cream

½ banana

3 broccoli florets

1 thin slice of root ginger, peeled and chopped (about ¼ tsp)

½ pear, cored and chopped

1 tbsp lemon juice

½ tsp **MORINGA LEAF** powder, or **WHEATGRASS** powder or **GREEN SUPERFOOD BLEND**

Frozen banana blended with pear creates a sweet, smooth texture and helps to mask the flavour of the broccoli, giving you the benefits of a green smoothie in a palatable, fruity mix. Moringa leaf powder helps to improve the bio-availability of the nutrients in this drink.

Chop the banana and put it into a freezer bag. Exclude all the air, then seal and freeze overnight or until solid. Put the banana into a blender or food processor and add the remaining ingredients and 150ml/5fl oz/ scant ⅔ cup water. Blend until smooth and creamy. Serve immediately.

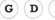 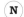 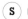

Nutritional information per serving
Kcals 81 | **Protein** 1.7g
Carbohydrates 16.9g, of which sugars 15.6g
Fat 0.3g, of which saturates 0.1g

½ banana

150ml/5fl oz/scant ⅔ cup cold **GREEN TEA**

½ pear, cored and chopped

½ kiwi fruit, peeled and chopped

1 handful of spinach leaves

¼ tsp **SPIRULINA** powder

¼ tsp **CAMU CAMU** powder, or **BAOBAB** powder or **ACAI BERRY** powder

Try this invigorating drink and you'll be hooked on the full flavour of spirulina. Green tea contains antioxidants to help fight free radicals, making this an anti-ageing drink.

Chop the banana and put it into a freezer bag. Exclude all the air, then seal and freeze overnight or until solid. Put the banana into a blender or food processor and add the remaining ingredients. Blend until smooth and creamy. Serve immediately.

Nutritional information per serving
Kcals 117 | **Protein** 3.8g
Carbohydrates 47.3g, of which sugars 18.1g
Fat 0.4g, of which saturates 0g

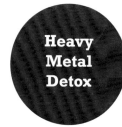

Heavy Metal Detox

Pictured>

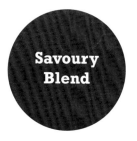

Savoury Blend

1 small banana
¼ tsp **CHLORELLA** powder
¼ tsp **WHEATGRASS** powder
1 tsp **GROUND FLAXSEED**
1 small handful of coriander leaves
1 small handful of watercress leaves
¼ mango, peeled and chopped
100ml/3½fl oz/generous ⅓ cup
   COCONUT WATER or water

Rich with coriander and watercress, and with fruity highlights, this intensely green smoothie packs quite a punch. It will keep your body clean and help to remove toxins and waste material – a great smoothie to include in a detox or cleansing programme. Freezing the banana keeps the taste fresh and light.

Chop the banana and put it into a freezer bag. Exclude all the air, then seal and freeze overnight or until solid. Put the banana into a blender or food processor and add the remaining ingredients. Blend until smooth and creamy. Serve immediately.

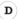   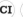 (V)

Nutritional information per serving
Kcals 142 | **Protein** 3g
Carbohydrates 27.9g, of which sugars 21.4g
Fat 1.9g, of which saturates 0.3g

2 tomatoes
3 tbsp **GOJI BERRIES**
½ red pepper, deseeded and chopped
½ cucumber, chopped
a pinch of Himalayan sea salt or sea salt
½ garlic clove, crushed (optional)
2 tsp **SHELLED HEMP SEEDS**
a few drops of Tabasco sauce or
   Worcestershire sauce, to taste
   (optional)
2 tbsp lemon juice
1 handful of parsley leaves, chopped
½ tsp **MACA** powder
100ml/3½fl oz/generous ⅓ cup
   COCONUT WATER

Give your immune system a lift with this light blend, rich in zinc and vitamins C and A. The optional garlic provides anti-microbial properties, and maca helps with stress, which depresses immunity.

Put all the ingredients into a blender or food processor and blend until smooth and creamy. Serve immediately.

Nutritional information per serving
Kcals 229 | **Protein** 6.6g
Carbohydrates 38.4g, of which sugars 30g
Fat 5.7g, of which saturates 0.4g

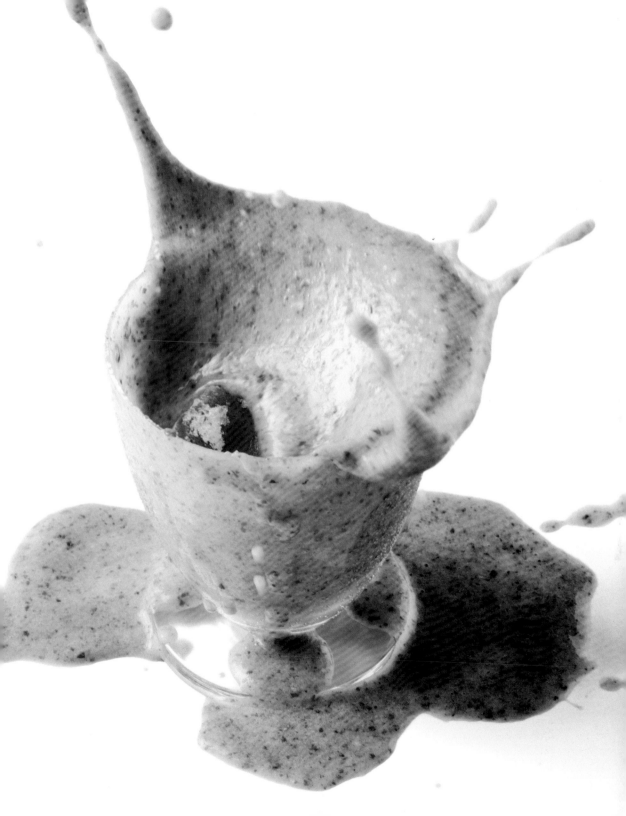

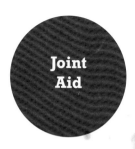

Joint Aid

½ mango, peeled and cut into chunks
60g/2¼oz/¼ cup tinned **pumpkin purée**, or sweet potato, steamed and mashed
1 pitted soft dried date
a pinch of ground cinnamon
¼ tsp ground **TURMERIC**
2 tsp **COLLAGEN** powder
1 tsp **GROUND FLAXSEED**
5mm/¼in piece of root ginger, peeled and grated
1 tbsp **GLUTAMINE** powder
½ tsp **MSM** powder
¼ tsp **BAOBAB** powder
150ml/5fl oz/scant ⅔ cup chilled herbal tea, **GREEN TEA or MATCHA GREEN TEA**
4 ice cubes or **COCONUT ICE CUBES** (page 22)

If you're suffering with aching joints, inflammation or stiffness, sip this luxurious-
tasting smoothie. It is also ideal as a beautifying tonic, being rich in skin-feeding
vitamin A, collagen and sulphur. For an antioxidant kick, I have added a little baobab
powder. If you like it a bit more spicy, increase the ginger.

Put all the ingredients, except the ice, into a blender or food processor and blend until
smooth and creamy. Add the ice and blend briefly to retain some texture. Serve immediately.

Nutritional information per serving
Kcals 198 | **Protein** 23.7g
Carbohydrates 57.2g, of which sugars 15.6g
Fat 1.7g, of which saturates 0.3g

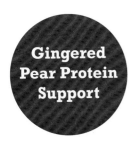

Gingered Pear Protein Support

2 tbsp **VANILLA PEA** or **HEMP PROTEIN POWDER**
½ tsp vanilla extract (optional)
5mm/¼in piece of root ginger, peeled and grated
1 pear, cored and chopped
1 tsp **COCONUT OIL**
1 tbsp **DRIED MULBERRIES** or **GOJI BERRIES**
1 tbsp **LUCUMA** powder
150ml/5fl oz/scant ⅔ cup **COCONUT WATER**

Tangy and energizing, this shake contains protein powder to promote healthy blood sugar levels as well as aiding the repair of muscles after a workout. Coconut oil is an excellent training fuel, because the body burns it for energy rather than storing it as fat. Lucuma is a natural caramel-flavoured sweetener.

Put all the ingredients into a blender or food processor and blend until smooth and creamy. Serve immediately.

(G) (D) (S) (SE) (CI) (V)

Nutritional information per serving
Kcals 281 | **Protein** 17.2g
Carbohydrates 36.3g, of which sugars 16.8g
Fat 7g, of which saturates 2.6g

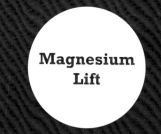

Magnesium Lift

½ **banana**
¼ **ripe avocado, peeled and chopped**
1 **small handful of spinach**
1 **handful of frozen berries**
1½ tsp **SHELLED HEMP SEEDS**
½ tsp **WHEATGRASS powder**
¼ **cucumber, chopped**
1 tbsp **RAW CACAO NIBS**
200ml/7fl oz/scant 1 cup **COCONUT WATER** or water, plus extra if needed

Although essential for energy production, magnesium is commonly low in people's diets, especially athletes. This creamy and hydrating mix will help to improve magnesium levels and it is also especially rich in electrolytes, potassium and sodium. The addition of wheatgrass powder adds an alkalizing punch to refresh and revitalize the body.

Chop the banana and put it into a freezer bag. Exclude all the air, then seal and freeze overnight or until solid. Put the banana into a blender or food processor and add the remaining ingredients. Blend until smooth and creamy, adding a little more water, if needed. Serve immediately.

Health Benefits

The range of nutrients in raw cacao includes exceptionally high levels of magnesium, iron, chromium and antioxidants. Cacao nibs contain no sugar but provide a natural feel-good lift, thanks to the chemicals contained in them, including tryptophan and phenylethylamine (PEA). PEA is the chemical produced in the brain associated with experiencing 'runner's high' and feelings of being in love. It helps to stimulate alertness and focus, producing an overall sense of well-being.

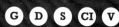

Nutritional information per serving
Kcals 257 | **Protein** 8.1g
Carbohydrates 25.5g, of which sugars 10.6g
Fat 15.2g, of which saturates 5g

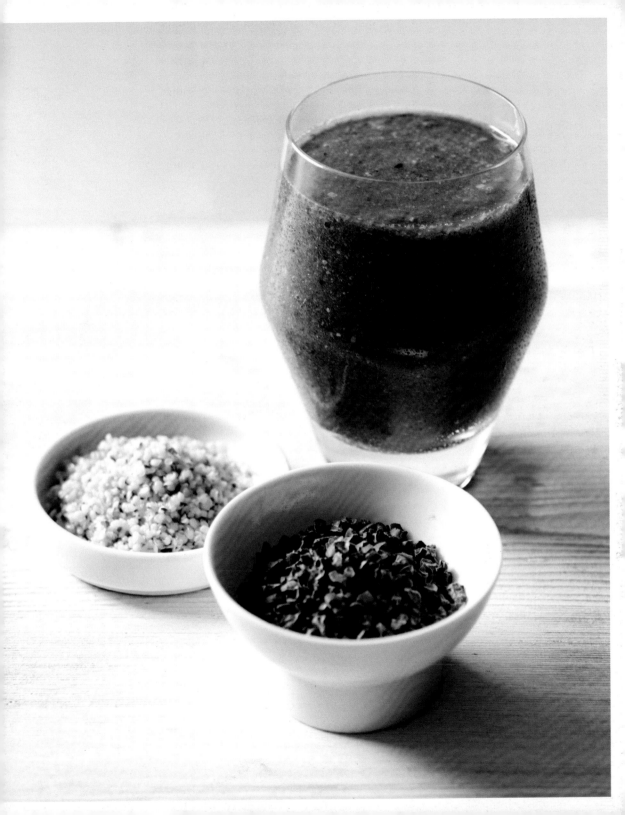

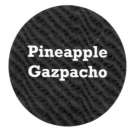

Matcha Green Tropical Blend

Pineapple Gazpacho

80g/2¾oz mango
80g/2¾oz pineapple
1 handful of romaine or cos lettuce leaves
¼ tsp MATCHA GREEN TEA powder
¼ tsp WHEATGRASS powder
125ml/4fl oz/½ cup COCONUT WATER
   or water
½ tsp CHIA SEEDS
2 tsp GOJI BERRIES
1 tbsp DRIED MULBERRIES (optional)
½ passion fruit, pulp and seeds only
4 ice cubes or COCONUT ICE CUBES
   (page 22)

Tropical fruits with supergreens.

Chop the mango and pineapple and put
them into a freezer bag. Exclude all the
air, then seal and freeze overnight or until
solid. Put the frozen fruit into a blender
or food processor and add the remaining
ingredients except the ice. Blend until
smooth and creamy. Add the ice and blend
briefly to combine. Serve immediately.

    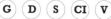

Nutritional information per serving
Kcals 153 | **Protein** 4.4g
Carbohydrates 30.6g, of which sugars 24.2g
Fat 1.6g, of which saturates 0.2g

½ cucumber, chopped
¼ pineapple, skin cut off, flesh chopped
1 tsp lime juice
1 small handful of coriander leaves
1 small handful of mint leaves
½ tsp WHEATGRASS powder
½ tsp COCONUT OIL
4 ice cubes or COCONUT ICE CUBES
   (page 22)

Herb leaves blend with pineapple and
cucumber to create a light and fruity
meal in a glass, which is iced to make it
super-refreshing for hot days. Wheatgrass
powder – a green supercharged food –
supplements the smoothie to increase its
cleansing properties further.

Put all the ingredients, except the ice, into a
blender or food processor and blend until
smooth and creamy. Add the ice and blend
briefly to retain some texture. Serve the
smoothie immediately.

Nutritional information per serving
Kcals 91 | **Protein** 1.6g
Carbohydrates 16.1g, of which sugars 15.4g
Fat 1.9g, of which saturates 1.3g

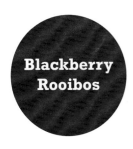

**Blackberry
Rooibos**

200ml/7fl oz/scant 1 cup chilled rooibos tea
60g/2¼oz/½ cup blackberries
30g/1oz/¼ cup blueberries
½ tsp **ACAI BERRY** powder
1 tbsp **DRIED MULBERRIES** or **GOJI BERRIES**
1 tsp **GROUND FLAXSEED**
½ small banana
½ tsp **FLAXSEED OIL**
1 handful of ice or **COCONUT ICE CUBES** (page 22)

**The tartness of the rooibos tea complements the sweet blackberries and blueberries
in this light and refreshing combination. Not only is rooibos caffeine-free but it is also
high in antioxidants. These qualities make it a nourishing base for smoothies.**

Put all the ingredients, except the ice, into a blender or food processor and blend until
smooth and creamy. Add the ice and blend briefly to retain some texture. Serve immediately.

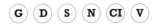

Nutritional information per serving
Kcals 111 | **Protein** 2.1g
Carbohydrates 15.9g, of which sugars 14.1g
Fat 4.2g, of which saturates 0.3g

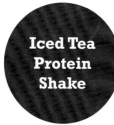

Iced Tea Protein Shake

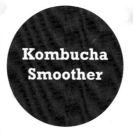

Kombucha Smoother

90g/3¼oz/½ cup frozen pitted cherries
100ml/3½fl oz/generous ⅓ cup cooled
  GREEN TEA
2 tbsp VANILLA PROTEIN powder
1 tsp ACAI BERRY powder
⅛ tsp CAMU CAMU powder or BAOBAB
  powder
2 tsp COLOSTRUM powder or
  GLUTAMINE powder
4 ice cubes or COCONUT ICE CUBES
  (page 22)

Cool down after a hard workout with this protein-packed shake. Cherries, plus antioxidant-rich superberry powders and colostrum make a winning formula. The balance of protein and carbs refuels and supports muscle recovery. Antioxidant-rich green tea is a natural fat burner.

Put all the ingredients, except the ice, into a blender or food processor and blend until smooth and creamy. Add the ice and blend briefly to retain some texture. Serve the smoothie immediately.

G S N SE CI

Nutritional information per serving
Kcals 213 | **Protein** 19.3g
Carbohydrates 45.2g, of which sugars 9.9g
Fat 5.4g, of which saturates 0g

½ banana
125ml/4fl oz/½ cup KOMBUCHA
  (page 22) or WATER KEFIR (page 22)
½ mango, peeled and chopped
juice of ½ lemon
5mm/¼in piece of root ginger, peeled
  and grated
1 tsp CHIA SEEDS
4 ice cubes

Kombucha is energizing and a great gut healer. It supports immune health, lowers inflammation and is a good source of antioxidants. The chia seeds provide essential omega-3 fats and protein.

Chop the banana and put it into a freezer bag. Exclude all the air, then seal and freeze overnight or until solid. Put the banana into a blender or food processor and add the remaining ingredients except the ice. Blend until smooth and creamy. Add the ice and blend to create a slushy drink. Serve the smoothie immediately.

G D S N V

Nutritional information per serving
Kcals 157 | **Protein** 2g
Carbohydrates 33.8g, of which sugars 31.5g
Fat 1.6g, of which saturates 0.3g

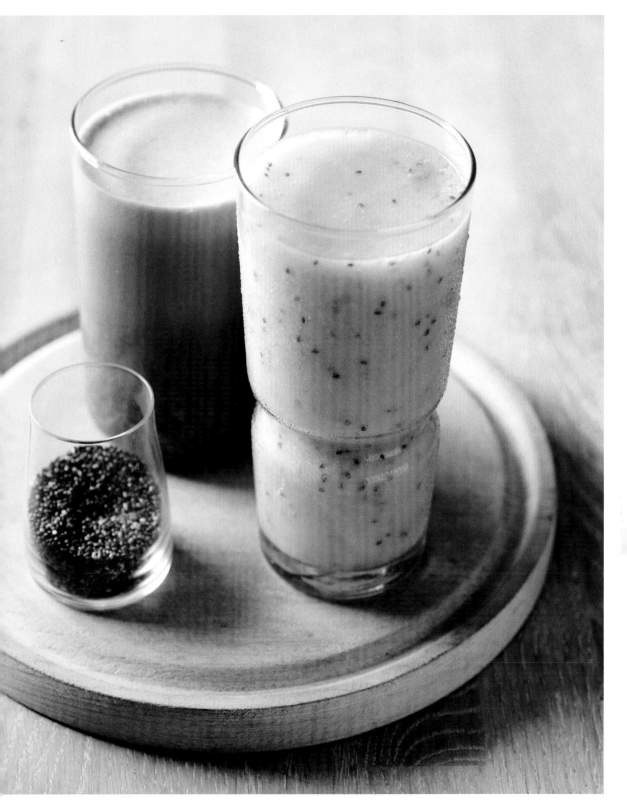

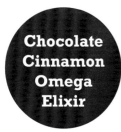

Chocolate Cinnamon Omega Elixir

2 tsp COCONUT OIL, melted
2–3 tsp RAW CACAO powder, to taste
1 tsp RAW CACAO NIBS
½ tsp MACA powder
½ tsp ground cinnamon
2 tbsp cashew nuts
1 tbsp GOJI BERRIES
1 tsp OMEGA OIL BLEND or
   FLAXSEED OIL
1 tsp MANUKA or RAW HONEY, or
   coconut syrup
2 tbsp PROTEIN powder
250ml/9fl oz/1 cup SCHIZANDRA TEA,
   hot or cooled

You can enjoy this rich and nourishing chocolate drink warm or cold. Traditionally used as a stress tonic and longevity herb, schizandra is considered to be a superb beauty tonic and to help improve brain and mental function.

Put all the ingredients into a blender or food processor and blend until smooth and creamy. Serve immediately.

Nutritional information per serving
Kcals 479 | **Protein** 23.5g
Carbohydrates 35.8g, of which sugars 16.6g
Fat 27.5g, of which saturates 9.7g

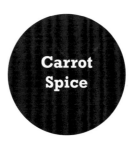

Carrot Spice

½ small banana
200ml/7fl oz/scant 1 cup carrot juice
   (about 5 carrots juiced)
1 tbsp GOJI BERRIES
1 apricot, pitted
½ tsp ground cinnamon
1 tbsp cashew nuts
80ml/2½fl oz/⅓ cup COCONUT WATER
a pinch of ground cardamom

This luscious smoothie takes the humble carrot juice to a new and tasty level. The combination of carrots and fruit creates a flavoursome sweet-tasting smoothie packed with skin- and immune-boosting beta-carotene, and vitamins A and C. The warming cinnamon helps to balance the blood sugar level.

Chop the banana and put it into a freezer bag. Exclude all the air, then seal and freeze overnight or until solid. Put the banana into a blender or food processor and add the remaining ingredients. Blend until smooth and creamy. Serve immediately.

Nutritional information per serving
Kcals 259 | **Protein** 5.6g
Carbohydrates 40.1g, of which sugars 33.5g
Fat 8.7g, of which saturates 1.5g

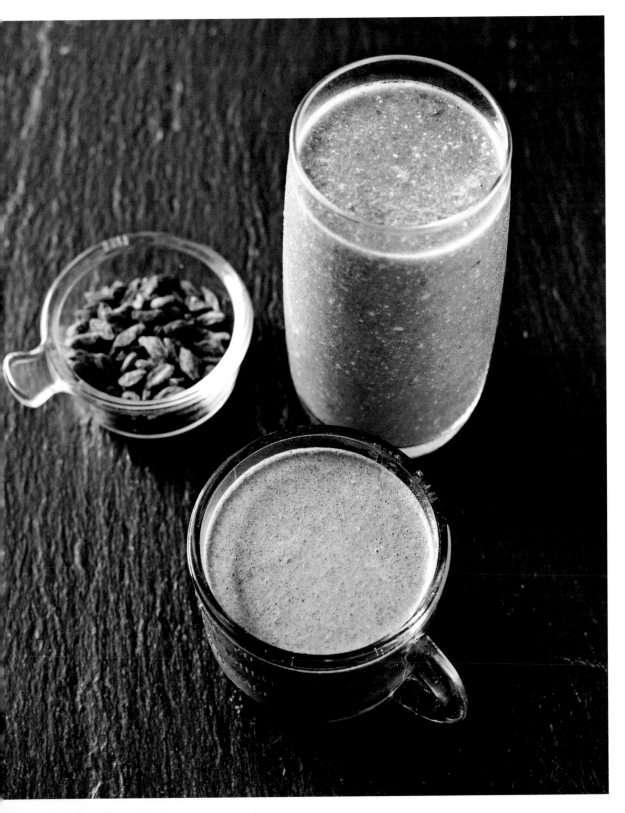

Chocolate Berry

1 small banana
1–1½ tbsp RAW CACAO powder, to taste
1½ tsp SHELLED HEMP SEEDS
90g/3¼oz/⅓ cup frozen mixed berries
2 tsp DRIED MULBERRIES or GOJI BERRIES
1 tsp GOJI BERRIES
½ tsp vanilla extract
¼ tsp CAMU CAMU powder or BAOBAB powder (optional)
½ tsp ACAI BERRY powder or MAQUI BERRY powder

The combination of berries and raw cacao powder tastes divine. This supercharged blend is high in antioxidants, vitamins and minerals, and the addition of hemp seeds provides beneficial essential fats too. Frozen banana makes the smoothie thick and inviting. For an additional supercharged burst add ¼ teaspoon superfood powder.

Chop the banana and put it into a freezer bag. Exclude all the air, then seal and freeze overnight or until solid. Put the banana into a blender or food processor and add the remaining ingredients and 200ml/7fl oz/scant 1 cup water. Blend until smooth and creamy. Serve immediately.

Health Benefits
Shelled hemp seeds have a temptingly creamy, mild and nutty flavour and are packed with easily digested protein, including all the essential amino acids to keep you energized. Rich in a wealth of minerals, including magnesium, calcium, potassium and sulphur, hemp is particularly known for its perfect 3:1 ratio of omega-6 to omega-3 essential fats, which nourish the body's cells and help to lower inflammation.

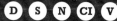

(G) (D) (S) (N) (CI) (V)

Nutritional information per serving
Kcals 240 | **Protein** 7.3g
Carbohydrates 65g, of which sugars 25.5g
Fat 4.5g, of which saturates 0.9g

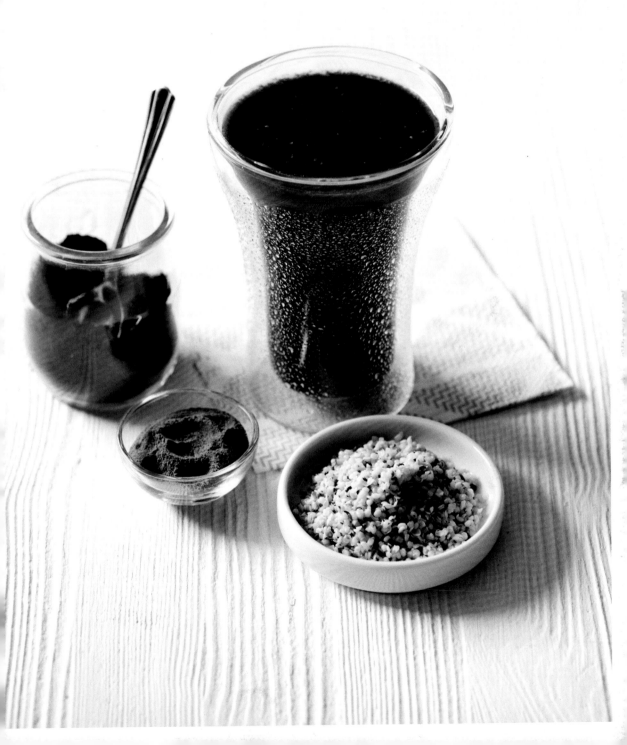

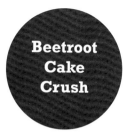

Beetroot Cake Crush

1 small beetroot
1 tbsp **RAW CACAO** powder
1 tbsp **GOJI BERRIES**
5 strawberries, stalks discarded
125ml/4fl oz/½ cup **WATER KEFIR** (page 22)
4 ice cubes or **COCONUT ICE CUBES** (page 22)
stevia, coconut sugar or xylitol (optional), to taste

If you're not a fan of beetroot, try adding this healthful vegetable to this chocolatey smoothie – which reminds me of beetroot chocolate cake. The raw cacao is a perfect partner for the sweet and smooth texture of roasted beetroot. When roasting the beetroot, it's worth cooking a few others at the same time to have hot as an accompanying vegetable with a meal or cold with salad. They will keep in the fridge for 3–4 days and freeze well too. Beetroots are a great source of phytonutrients, providing antioxidant, anti-inflammatory and detoxification support. They are also a source of betaine – a key body nutrient made from the B-complex vitamin, choline, which can help to regulate inflammation in the cardiovascular system.

Preheat the oven to 190°C/375°F/Gas 5. Wrap the beetroot in foil and roast for 1 hour or until softened when squeezed. Leave until cool enough to handle, then peel off the skin. Cut the beetroot in half and chop one half. Leave to cool. Keep the other half for another use.

Put the chopped beetroot and the remaining ingredients, except the ice and stevia, if using, into a blender or food processor and blend until smooth and creamy. Add the ice and blend to create a slushy drink. Sweeten to taste, if needed. Serve immediately.

(G) (D) (S) (N) (SE) (CI) (V)

Nutritional information per serving
Kcals 170 | **Protein** 3.4g
Carbohydrates 34.9g, of which sugars 25.9g
Fat 1.9g, of which saturates 0.6g

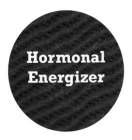

Hormonal Energizer

½ banana
1 handful of fresh or frozen blueberries
¼ tsp SPIRULINA powder
1 tsp MANUKA or RAW HONEY
½ tsp SHATAVARI powder (optional)
2 tsp LUCUMA powder
½ tsp OMEGA OIL BLEND or FLAXSEED OIL
1 tsp MACA powder
1 tbsp almond butter
1 tsp COCONUT OIL
150ml/5fl oz/scant ⅔ cup COCONUT WATER

If you have menopausal problems, PMS or low fertility, try this super-powered blend designed to balance the hormones and nourish the adrenal glands.

Chop the banana and put it into a freezer bag. Exclude all the air, then seal and freeze overnight or until solid. Put the banana into a blender or food processor and add the remaining ingredients. Blend until smooth and creamy. Serve immediately.

(G) (D) (S) (CI)

Nutritional information per serving
Kcals 313 | **Protein** 8.6g
Carbohydrates 59.6g, of which sugars 15.9g
Fat 15.3g, of which saturates 3.8g

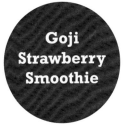

Goji Strawberry Smoothie

½ small banana
1 tbsp GOJI BERRIES
150ml/5fl oz/scant ⅔ cup COCONUT WATER
1 tsp CHIA SEEDS
1 tsp SHELLED HEMP SEEDS
1 handful of strawberries, stalks discarded, chopped
2 tbsp VANILLA PROTEIN powder

Start the day with this protein-rich, energy-boosting smoothie. It's best to soak the goji berries in the coconut water, if you have time, to allow them to plump up and be easily combined.

Chop the banana and put it into a freezer bag. Exclude all the air, then seal and freeze overnight or until solid. Soak the goji berries in the coconut water for 10 minutes. Put the banana, goji berries and coconut water into a blender or food processor and add the remaining ingredients. Blend until smooth and creamy. Serve immediately.

(G) (S) (CI)

Nutritional information per serving
Kcals 285 | **Protein** 18.9g
Carbohydrates 37.4g, of which sugars 23.2g
Fat 6.7g, of which saturates 0.2g

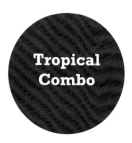

Tropical Combo

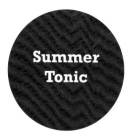

Summer Tonic

80g/2¾oz pineapple, chopped
2 lychees, tinned or fresh, pitted
¼ papaya, peeled, deseeded and chopped
½ tsp MACA powder
1 tbsp desiccated coconut
1 tbsp DRIED MULBERRIES or GOJI BERRIES
1 tsp LUCUMA powder
1 tbsp COLLAGEN powder
2 tsp COLOSTRUM powder or GLUTAMINE powder
150ml/5fl oz/scant ⅔ cup COCONUT WATER or water

With exotic fruits to bring you thoughts of sunny climes, this smoothie will energize your body and nourish your immune system. Colostrum improves immune function and aids gut health, while collagen provides support to the joints, bones and skin.

Put all the ingredients into a blender or food processor and blend until smooth and creamy. Serve immediately.

Nutritional information per serving
Kcals 259 | **Protein** 19.2g
Carbohydrates 26.5g, of which sugars 14.1g
Fat 9g, of which saturates 6.9g

90g/3¼oz cantaloupe melon, flesh chopped
2 peaches, pitted and chopped
¼ tsp BAOBAB powder
2 tsp LUCUMA powder
1 tsp lime zest
juice of ½ lime
¼ tsp CAMU CAMU powder or ACAI BERRY powder
1 tbsp GOJI BERRIES
2 tbsp VANILLA or PLAIN PROTEIN powder
½ tsp vanilla extract
150ml/5fl oz/scant ⅔ cup COCONUT WATER or water
4 ice cubes

For a lean, toned body, try this protein-packed and antioxidant-rich smoothie, with vitamin C-rich fruits and powders.

Put all the ingredients, except the ice, into a blender or food processor and blend until smooth and creamy. Add the ice and blend to create a slushy drink. Serve immediately.

 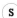

Nutritional information per serving
Kcals 285 | **Protein** 19.2g
Carbohydrates 64.7g, of which sugars 26g
Fat 4.6g, of which saturates 0g

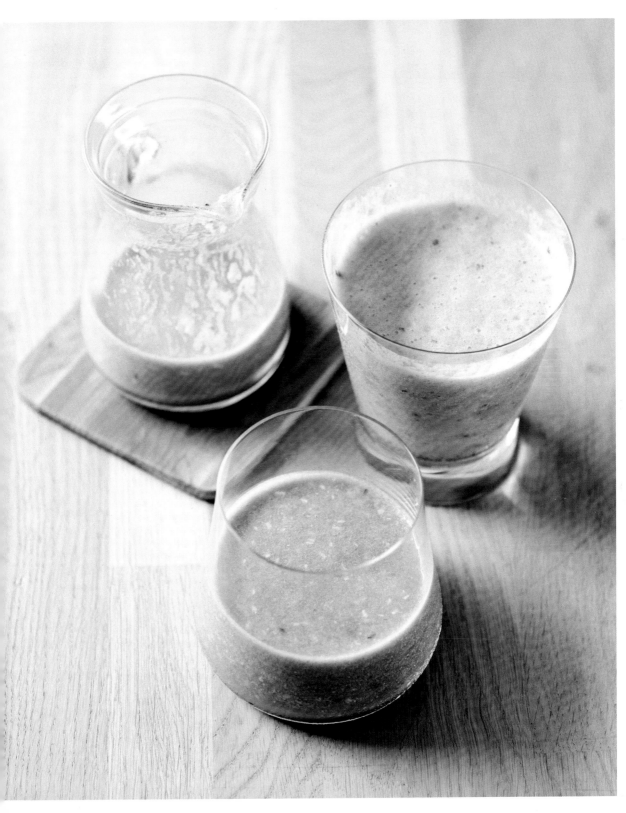

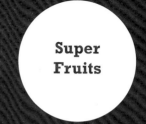

Super Fruits

150ml/5fl oz/scant ⅔ cup POMEGRANATE juice
½ pear, cored and chopped
1 small handful of mint leaves
2 tsp LUCUMA powder
90g/3¼oz/⅓ cup frozen mixed berries
1 tsp lemon juice
¼ tsp CAMU CAMU powder or BAOBAB powder
½ tsp ACAI BERRY powder or MAQUI BERRY powder
1 tbsp GOJI BERRIES
4 ice cubes

A burst of berry goodness, this refreshing iced drink is an explosion of tart and sweet fruits. Blending in the goji berries increases the protein content and fibre as well as naturally thickening the juice. A handful of fresh mint brings lightness to the juice while it soothes the digestive tract and eases abdominal cramps.

Put all the ingredients, except the ice, into a blender or food processor and blend until smooth and creamy. Add the ice and blend briefly to retain some texture. Serve immediately.

Health Benefits
One of the easiest natural ways to boost your vitamin C intake is to add a little camu camu powder to your drinks. Camu camu contains the highest concentration of natural vitamin C than any other food, with around 2g of vitamin C per 100g/3½ oz of fruit. This means that you need only ¼ –½ teaspoon in smoothies for a real vitamin-C punch. Camu camu helps to support a healthy immune system and healthy skin, and it protects the body's cells, including the brain, from damage. Vitamin C is also essential for the formation of collagen, making this a superb choice for joint health.

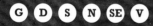

Nutritional information per serving
Kcals 231 | **Protein** 3g
Carbohydrates 48g, of which sugars 40g
Fat 2.7g, of which saturates 0.1g

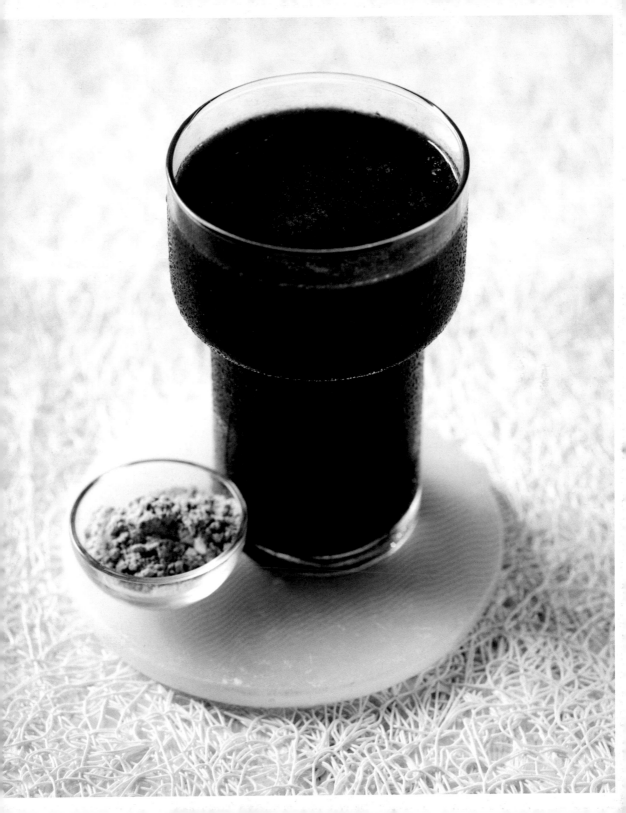

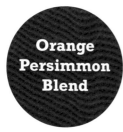

Orange Persimmon Blend

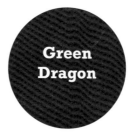

Green Dragon

1 persimmon (Sharon fruit), chopped
5mm/¼in piece of root ginger, peeled
   and chopped
½ tsp MACA powder
¼ tsp ground cinnamon
1 small handful of spinach or kale
1 orange, peeled
3 macadamia nuts (optional)
1 tbsp GOJI BERRIES

Sharon fruits, or persimmon, are an
excellent source of a number of nutrients:
soluble fibre to keep you feeling
energized; antioxidants, including eye-
protective carotenoids, such as lutein
and zeaxanthin; vitamin C; and energy-
promoting B vitamins. The macadamia
nuts are optional, but they do add a
delicious silky texture to this drink.

Put all the ingredients into a blender or
food processor and blend until smooth and
creamy. Add a little water if needed to thin.
Serve immediately.

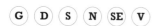

Nutritional information per serving
Kcals 191 | **Protein** 3.1g
Carbohydrates 30.6g, of which sugars 28.3g
Fat 6.5g, of which saturates 0.8g

½ banana
½ dragon fruit, peeled and chopped
2 tbsp desiccated coconut
1 handful of pak choi leaves or
   spinach leaves
½ tsp WHEATGRASS powder
200ml/7fl oz/scant 1 cup COCONUT
   WATER

The flavour of the exotic dragon fruit
resembles a cross between a kiwi and
pear. It is relatively low in calories yet
packed with vitamin C and a good source
of calcium too. I have blended it here with
greens and wheatgrass powder to create
a tasty yet cleansing blend.

Chop the banana and put it into a freezer
bag. Exclude all the air, then seal and freeze
overnight or until solid. Put the banana into
a blender or food processor and add the
remaining ingredients. Blend until smooth
and creamy. Serve immediately.

(G) (D) (S) (SE) (CI) (V)

Nutritional information per serving
Kcals 201 | **Protein** 4.2g
Carbohydrates 21.5g, of which sugars 9.1g
Fat 10.6g, of which saturates 8.1g

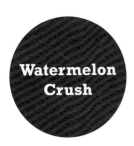

Watermelon Crush

150g/5½oz/1 cup strawberries, stalks discarded, chopped
160g/5¾oz watermelon flesh
1 tsp **CHIA SEEDS**
a few drops of stevia or a little coconut sugar, to taste
1 tsp lime zest
juice of ½ lime
¼ tsp **BAOBAB** powder
4 ice cubes or **COCONUT ICE CUBES** (page 22)

An array of antioxidants contained in this hydrating summer drink make it beneficial for nourishing the skin and protecting it from sun damage. Watermelon is also one of the richest sources of lycopene, a carotenoid that has been shown to be important for cardiovascular and bone health. Chia seeds thicken the smoothie as well as adding valuable omega-3 fats and protein.

Put all the ingredients into a blender or food processor and blend until smooth and creamy. Serve immediately.

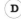

Nutritional information per serving
Kcals 167 | **Protein** 6.4g
Carbohydrates 77.7g, of which sugars 18.9g
Fat 1.9g, of which saturates 0.3g

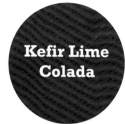

Kefir Lime Colada

Pictured>

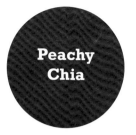

Peachy Chia

zest and juice of 1 lime
80g/2¾oz fresh or frozen pineapple, chopped
1 tbsp LUCUMA powder
250ml/9fl oz/1 cup WATER KEFIR (page 22)
1 tsp TOCOTRIENOLS or oil of 1 vitamin E capsule, plus the squeezed capsule
1 tsp PROBIOTIC powder
1 tsp MANUKA or RAW HONEY, or coconut sugar
4 ice cubes

Water kefir is simple to make and an effective way to support your gut health and give your immune system a boost as well. By blending in fruit and supercharged foods you create an amazing, healthy, fizzy smoothie.

Put all the ingredients, except the ice, into a blender or food processor and blend until smooth and creamy. Add the ice and blend to create a slushy drink. Serve immediately.

  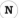 G S N SE

Nutritional information per serving
Kcals 177 | **Protein** 1.5g
Carbohydrates 41.2g, of which sugars 32.4g
Fat 0.2g, of which saturates 0g

2 tsp CHIA SEEDS
170ml/5½fl oz/⅔ cup COCONUT WATER
1 peach, pitted and chopped
1 handful of fresh or frozen raspberries
¼ tsp MAQUI BERRY powder (optional)
1 tsp ACAI BERRY powder
1 tsp lemon juice
¼ tsp ground cinnamon

Chia seeds supply soluble fibre and omega-3 fats to this thick smoothie with its fruity sweetness from peach and raspberries. Take this drink to stabilize your blood sugar level and keep you feeling full and satisfied. The berry powders gives this shake a tremendous antioxidant and vitamin C boost.

Put the chia seeds in a bowl and add the coconut water. Stir well, then leave for 10 minutes to allow the seeds to swell up. Transfer to a blender or food processor and add the remaining ingredients. Blend until smooth and creamy. Serve immediately.

   G D S V

Nutritional information per serving
Kcals 114 | **Protein** 3.4g
Carbohydrates 16.6g, of which sugars 6.7g
Fat 3.9g, of which saturates 0.2g

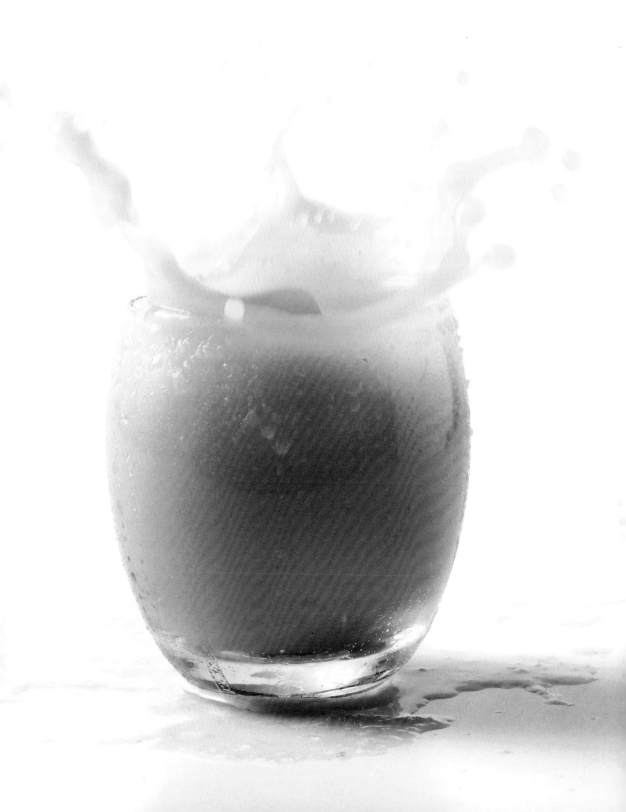

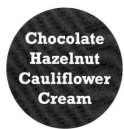

Chocolate Hazelnut Cauliflower Cream

½ banana
90g/3¼oz/¾ cup cauliflower florets
1 tbsp hazelnuts
200ml/7fl oz/scant 1 cup COCONUT
  WATER, plus extra if needed
1 tbsp RAW CACAO powder
1 tsp vanilla extract
½ tsp ground cinnamon
2 tsp LUCUMA powder
2 pitted soft dried dates

Health-promoting cauliflower creates a lovely velvety texture to this drink.

Chop the banana and put it into a freezer bag. Add the cauliflower florets. Exclude all the air, then seal and freeze overnight or until solid. Put the hazelnuts in a frying pan and toast over a medium heat until golden. Cool. Put the hazelnuts and coconut water into a blender or food processor and blend until smooth. Add the banana, cauliflower and the remaining ingredients, and blend until smooth and creamy. Add a little more coconut water to thin if needed. Serve.

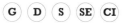

Nutritional information per serving
Kcals 287 | **Protein** 9.9g
Carbohydrates 34.7g, of which sugars 14.1g
Fat 11.9g, of which saturates 1.5g

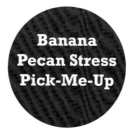

Banana Pecan Stress Pick-Me-Up

1 banana
4 pitted soft dried dates
1 tsp COCONUT OIL, melted
2 tbsp pecan nuts
1 tsp SHELLED HEMP SEEDS
1 tsp MACA powder
250ml/9fl oz/1 cup cold LIQUORICE
  or GINSENG TEA
2 tsp vanilla extract
a pinch of sea salt

Pecan nuts create a rich, milky texture for smoothies. Try this energizing drink on stressful days to give you a natural lift. Liquorice or ginseng tea and maca are all known adaptogens enabling the body to cope more efficiently with stress and supporting healthy adrenal function.

Chop the banana and put it into a freezer bag. Exclude all the air, then seal and freeze overnight or until solid. Put the banana into a blender or food processor and add the remaining ingredients. Blend until smooth and creamy. Serve immediately.

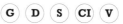

Nutritional information per serving
Kcals 360 | **Protein** 5.4g
Carbohydrates 27g, of which sugars 25.2g
Fat 25.6g, of which saturates 4.5g

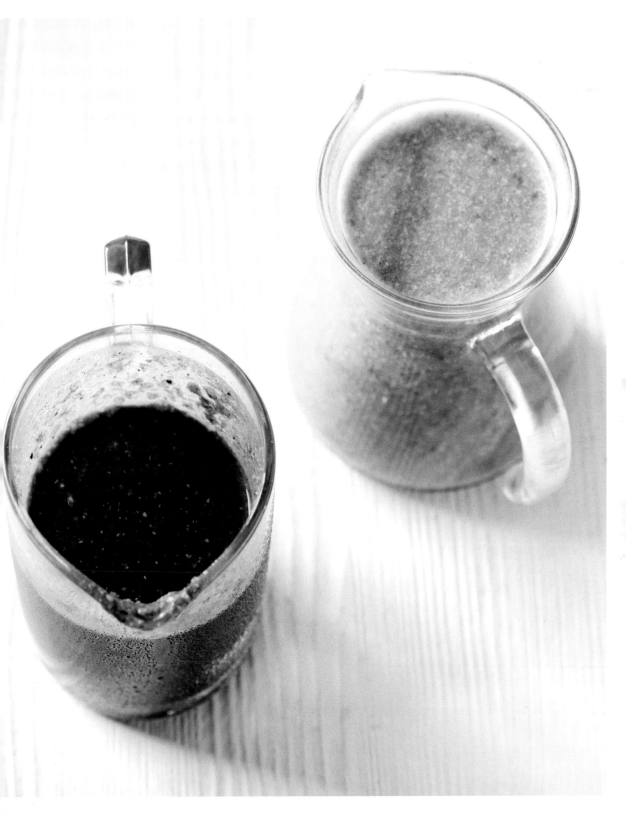

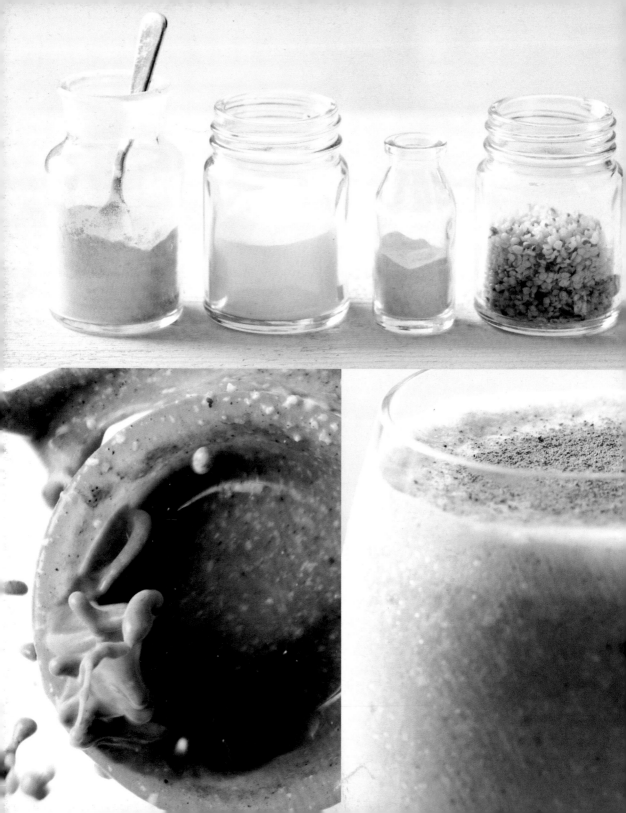

CHAPTER 4

CREAMY SMOOTHIES

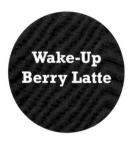

Wake-Up Berry Latte

Kick-Start

1 yerbe mate tea bag, or 1½ tbsp loose tea
    or 1 tsp instant coffee/coffee alternative
150ml/5fl oz/scant ⅔ cup almond milk
½ tsp **MAQUI BERRY** powder or
    ACAI BERRY powder
100g/3½oz/½ cup frozen mixed berries
½ tsp ground cinnamon

Think clearer and stay more focused
throughout the day with this latte.
Yerbe mate tea is a good alternative to
coffee, because it is lower in caffeine
and can give you a clean caffeine-like
buzz without the jitters. Plus, it contains
antioxidants, vitamins and minerals.

At night, put the tea in a jug and pour over
100ml/3½fl oz/generous ⅓ cup hot (not
boiling) water. Leave to infuse for 20 minutes
or longer if you prefer a stronger brew.
Strain and chill overnight. Next morning,
put the tea and the remaining ingredients
into a blender or food processor and blend
until smooth and creamy. Serve immediately.

(G) (D) (S) (SE) (CI) (V)

Nutritional information per serving
Kcals 82 | **Protein** 1g
Carbohydrates 13.1g, of which sugars 6.6g
Fat 2.7g, of which saturates 0g

1 small banana
3 ready-to-eat pitted prunes
2 tsp **GROUND FLAXSEED**
2 tsp **RAW CACAO** powder
2 tsp **RAW CACAO NIBS**
1 tbsp **HEMP PROTEIN** powder
250ml/9fl oz/1 cup almond milk
4 Brazil nuts
1 tsp **PROBIOTIC** powder

Here is a supercharged smoothie infusion
well supplied with fibre, protein and
omega-3 fats to give you an energizing
start to the day. A spoonful of probiotic
powder is included to help settle ongoing
digestive problems, and the prunes and
flaxseed can tackle constipation.

Chop the banana and put it into a freezer
bag. Exclude all the air, then seal and freeze
overnight or until solid. Put the banana into
a blender or food processor and add the
remaining ingredients. Blend until smooth
and creamy. Serve immediately.

(G) (S) (CI)

Nutritional information per serving
Kcals 386 | **Protein** 13.9g
Carbohydrates 42.3g, of which sugars 22.1g
Fat 18.3g, of which saturates 4.1g

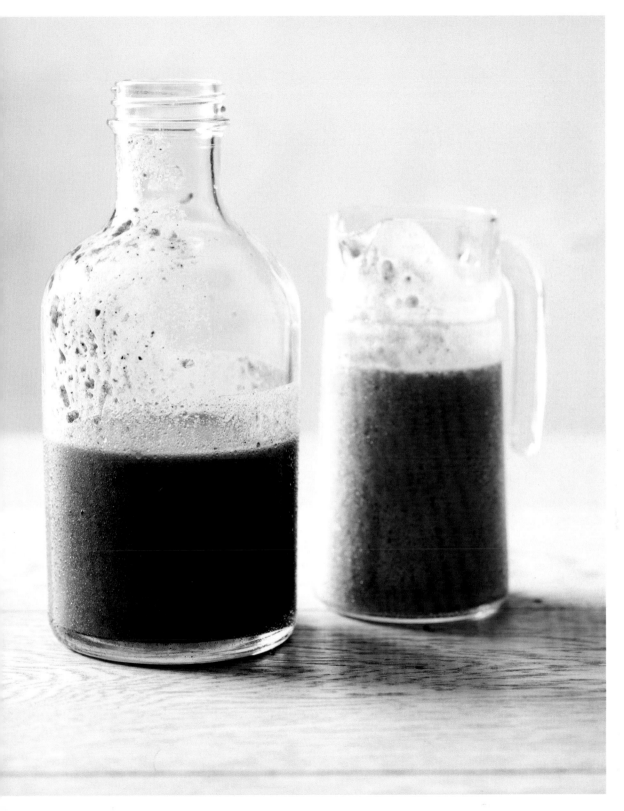

½ tsp GREEN SUPERFOOD BLEND or
   WHEATGRASS powder
2 tsp RAW CACAO powder
2 pitted soft dried dates
1 tsp MACA powder
1 tbsp almond butter
½ tsp CAMU CAMU powder, or BAOBAB powder
   or ACAI BERRY powder
2 tsp LUCUMA powder
½ tsp vanilla extract
¼ tsp ground cinnamon
1 tsp SHELLED HEMP SEEDS
125ml/4fl oz/½ cup prepared chicory or dandelion coffee
100ml/3½fl oz/generous ⅓ cup COCONUT WATER
1 tbsp RAW CACAO NIBS
4–5 ice cubes or COCONUT ICE CUBES (page 22)

Tasting richly of coffee and chocolate, this smoothie is a supercharged special. It contains maca for those days when you are feeling stressed, supporting the adrenal glands and giving you a natural lift. Although you could use coffee, I have chosen a coffee substitute known as chicory root – a great source of prebiotics to keep the gut healthy – but dandelion coffee would also work well.

Put all the ingredients, except the cacao nibs and ice, into a blender or food processor and blend until smooth and creamy. Add the cacao nibs and ice, and blend briefly to retain some texture. Serve immediately.

Health Benefits
Chicory has a long history of health benefits for the liver and digestion. Chicory root is thought to increase the flow of bile, which supports digestion and emulsification of fats. Being rich in inulin, a soluble fibre that feeds healthy bacteria, it can help with digestive health. Soluble fibre is also great for stabilizing blood sugar, making it useful for weight loss.

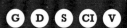

Nutritional information per serving
Kcals 308 | **Protein** 11.7g
Carbohydrates 51.6g, of which sugars 4.2g
Fat 18.9g, of which saturates 5.2g

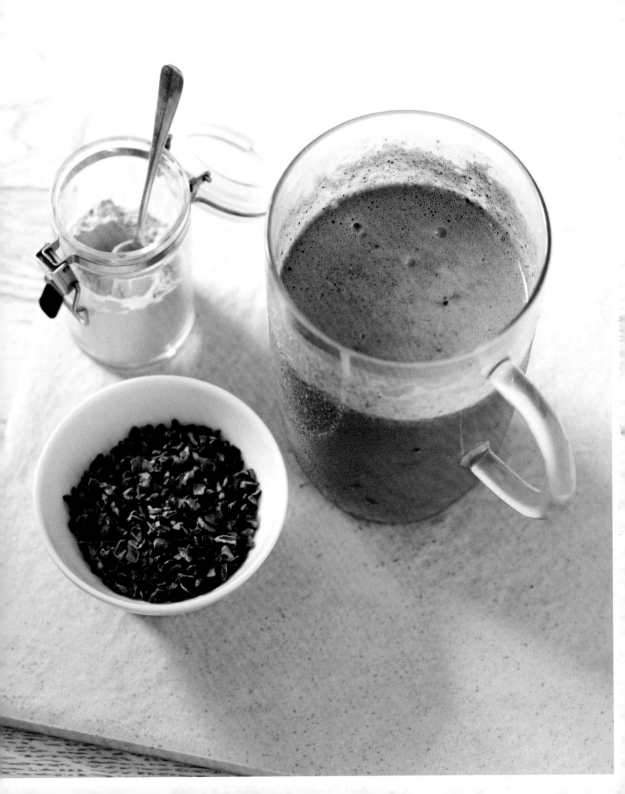

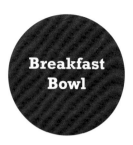

Breakfast Bowl

1 tbsp porridge oats
1 tbsp desiccated coconut
3 macadamia nuts, chopped
1 tsp pumpkin seeds
1 tsp GROUND FLAXSEED
½ tsp ground cinnamon
1 handful fresh or frozen strawberries, stalks discarded if fresh
1 tbsp lime juice
1 tbsp GOJI BERRIES
100ml/3½fl oz/generous ⅓ cup natural yogurt or soya yogurt
150ml/5fl oz/scant ⅔ cup semi-skimmed milk or milk alternative

Smoothies are a great way to start the day, but sometimes you need something more substantial. This thicker-than-normal smoothie really is breakfast in a glass. It has a crunchy oat topping made with slow-releasing carbohydrates to help keep you focused throughout the morning. Oats and strawberries are rich in B vitamins, essential for energy and to support the body during times of stress.

Heat a non-stick frying pan over a medium heat and gently toast the oats, coconut, macadamia nuts and pumpkin seeds for 2–3 minutes until lightly golden. Pour into a bowl and stir in the flaxseed and cinnamon.

Put the remaining ingredients into a blender or food processor and blend until smooth and creamy. Add half the oat mixture and blend again. Pour into glasses and top with the remaining oat mixture, or stir it in if you prefer. Serve immediately and eat with a spoon.

Nutritional information per serving
Kcals 486 | **Protein** 16.3g
Carbohydrates 44.6g, of which sugars 32.7g
Fat 27g, of which saturates 9.8g

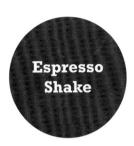

Espresso Shake

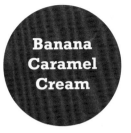

Banana Caramel Cream

1 small banana, unpeeled
250ml/9fl oz/1 cup full-fat coconut milk
1 tbsp almond butter
¼ tsp ground cinnamon
1 tbsp LUCUMA powder
1 tsp MACA powder (optional)
1 tsp CHIA SEEDS
2 pitted soft dried dates

This sweet-tasting smoothie is based on roasted banana blended with dates and caramel-flavoured lucuma, making it as tasty as a dessert. Chia seeds provide omega-3 fats as well as soluble fibre.

Preheat the oven to 180°C/350°F/Gas 4. Put the unpeeled banana on a baking sheet and bake for 20 minutes or until the skin is blackened. Leave to cool, then peel off the skin.

Put the banana into a blender or food processor and add the remaining ingredients. Blend until smooth and creamy. Serve immediately.

 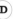

Nutritional information per serving
Kcals 308 | **Protein** 5.7g
Carbohydrates 46.2g, of which sugars 33.4g
Fat 11.7g, of which saturates 1.6g

2 pitted soft dried dates
2 tbsp VANILLA PROTEIN powder
1 tsp espresso coffee powder
1 tsp almond butter
200ml/7fl oz/scant 1 cup almond milk
  (page 21)
1 tsp SHELLED HEMP SEEDS
1 tsp CHIA SEEDS

Enjoy this caffeine boost pre-workout. The inclusion of protein powder and seeds helps to prevent your blood sugar fluctuating wildly, as well as providing you with lots of energy for training. If you like, you can also give the drink a mocha flavour by adding 1 tablespoon raw cacao powder to the mix.

Put all the ingredients into a blender or food processor and blend until smooth and creamy. Serve immediately.

Nutritional information per serving
Kcals 257 | **Protein** 18.6g
Carbohydrates 18.2g, of which sugars 2.7g
Fat 12.5g, of which saturates 0.6g

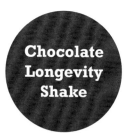

Chocolate Longevity Shake

4 Brazil nuts
1 tsp MACA powder
1 tbsp RAW CACAO powder
½ tsp MEDICINAL MUSHROOM powder
250ml/9fl oz/1 cup almond milk
    (page 21)
1 tsp MANUKA or RAW HONEY
½ tsp COCONUT OIL, melted
½ tsp vanilla extract
4 COCONUT ICE CUBES (page 22)
    or ice cubes

This vitalizing concoction is sublimely creamy with the addition of maca and cacao. For an additional healthy burst, add ¼ teaspoon green superfood powder.

Put all the ingredients, except the ice, into a blender or food processor and blend until smooth and creamy. Add the ice and blend briefly to retain some texture. Serve.

(G) (D) (S) (SE) (CI)

Nutritional information per serving
Kcals 250 | **Protein** 5.2g
Carbohydrates 22.8g, of which sugars 3.3g
Fat 15.2g, of which saturates 4.5g

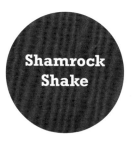

Shamrock Shake

1 tsp COCONUT OIL, melted
1 tsp almond butter
1 handful of spinach leaves
1 small handful of mint leaves
2 tbsp RAW CACAO NIBS
½ tsp TOCOTRIENOLS or 1 vitamin E
    capsule, plus the squeezed capsule
½ tsp vanilla extract
½ tsp GREEN SUPERFOOD powder,
    such as WHEATGRASS or CHLORELLA
250ml/9fl oz/1 cup almond milk
1 tsp MANUKA or RAW HONEY
4 ice cubes or COCONUT ICE CUBES
    (page 22)

Use any green superfood powder you have to hand. Wheatgrass will create a milder flavour whereas chlorella is ideal for a stronger shake. Tocotrienols contain vitamin E, proteins and minerals.

Put all the ingredients, except the ice, into a blender or food processor and blend until smooth and creamy. Add the ice and blend until incorporated. Serve immediately.

 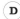

(G) (D) (S) (SE) (CI)

Nutritional information per serving
Kcals 217 | **Protein** 4.2g
Carbohydrates 19.7g, of which sugars 3.2g
Fat 15.3g, of which saturates 6.7g

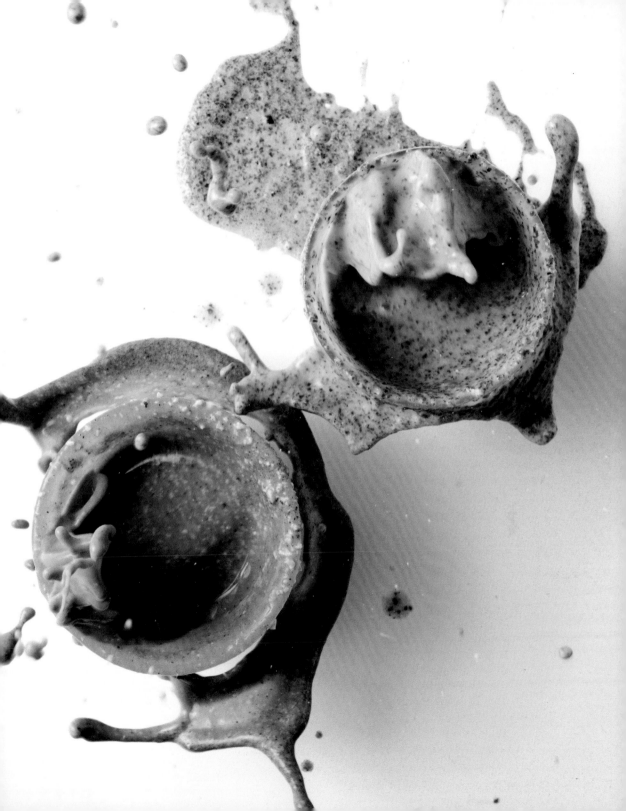

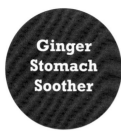

Ginger Stomach Soother

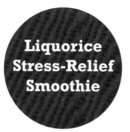

Liquorice Stress-Relief Smoothie

5mm/¼in piece of root ginger,
   peeled and grated
¼ papaya, peeled, deseeded and chopped
½ small mango, peeled and chopped
1 tbsp DRIED MULBERRIES or
   GOJI BERRIES
½ tsp PROBIOTIC powder
juice of ½ lime
1 tbsp unsweetened coconut flakes
2 tsp ALOE VERA juice
125ml/4fl oz/½ cup low-fat coconut milk
125ml/4fl oz/½ cup COCONUT WATER
   or water

Ginger has potent anti-microbial and
anti-inflammatory properties, which
are soothing for digestive upsets. The
gingerols contained in it are thought
to inhibit the growth of the bacterium
Helicobacter pylori, which is linked to
dyspepsia and stomach ulcers.

Put all the ingredients into a blender or
food processor and blend until smooth
and creamy. Serve immediately.

 (G) (S) (SE)

Nutritional information per serving
Kcals 198 | **Protein** 3.1g
Carbohydrates 24.6g, of which sugars 17.3g
Fat 9.6g, of which saturates 6g

2½ tbsp desiccated coconut
2 tbsp cashew nuts
200ml/7fl oz/scant 1 cup COCONUT
   WATER
4 strawberries, stalks discarded
¼ tsp LIQUORICE EXTRACT or powder
4 COCONUT ICE CUBES (page 22) or
   ice cubes

Coconut and liquorice combine to
make a rich, creamy and energizing
blend. Known as a stress-supporting
herb, liquorice also appears to
enhance immunity by boosting levels
of interferon, a key immune-system
chemical that fights off attacking viruses.
Use solid liquorice extract or the powder.

Put the coconut, cashew nuts and coconut
water into a blender or food processor
and blend until smooth and creamy. Add
the strawberries and liquorice extract, and
blend until smooth. Add the ice and blend
briefly to retain some texture. Serve.

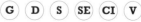 (G) (D) (S) (SE) (CI) (V)

Nutritional information per serving
Kcals 235 | **Protein** 5.7g
Carbohydrates 14.8g, of which sugars 4.3g
Fat 17g, of which saturates 9.4g

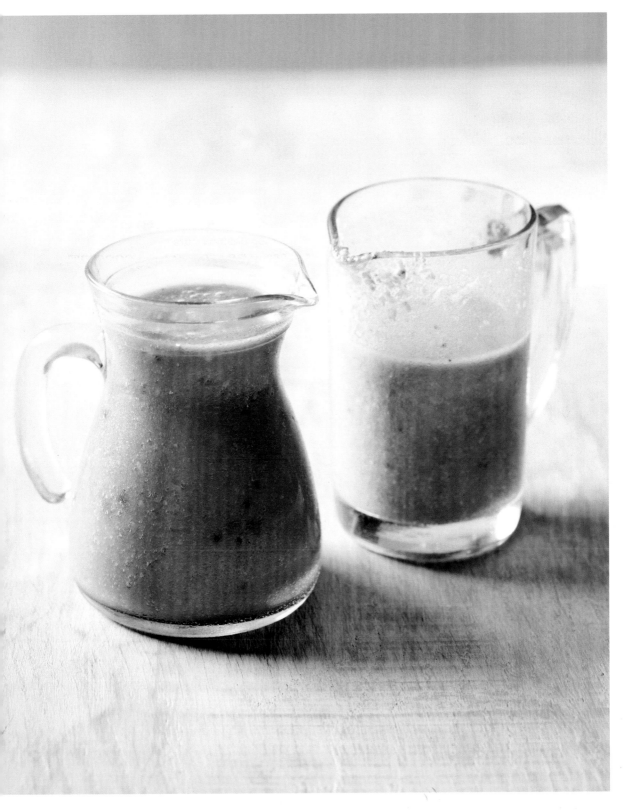

Joint-Health Greens

1 handful of kale leaves
½ papaya, peeled, deseeded and chopped
250ml/9fl oz/1 cup almond milk (page 21)
1 tsp almond butter
1 tbsp **HEMP PROTEIN** powder
½ tsp **WHEATGRASS** powder
1 tbsp **COLLAGEN** powder
1 tsp **CISSUS QUADRANGULARIS** powder or tincture

Greens, such as kale, contain alkalizing minerals that are important for healthy tissues and bones, and here they are blended with papaya to make a fruity smoothie. Almonds are one of the best sources of vitamin E, which protects the outer membrane of joint cells. Vitamin C in the fruit and kale, plus the addition of collagen, is beneficial for the connective tissue around the joints and, together with protein powder and the minerals calcium and magnesium in the kale and wheatgrass, it ensures healthy bone and joints. The health and strength of joints, cartilage and tendons are also aided by the herb Cissus quadrangularis, which is particularly important for people with osteoporosis or those who are recovering after injury.

Put all the ingredients into a blender or food processor and blend until smooth and creamy. Serve immediately.

Nutritional information per serving
Kcals 236 | **Protein** 22.6g
Carbohydrates 19g, of which sugars 0.5g
Fat 7.9g, of which saturates 0.3g

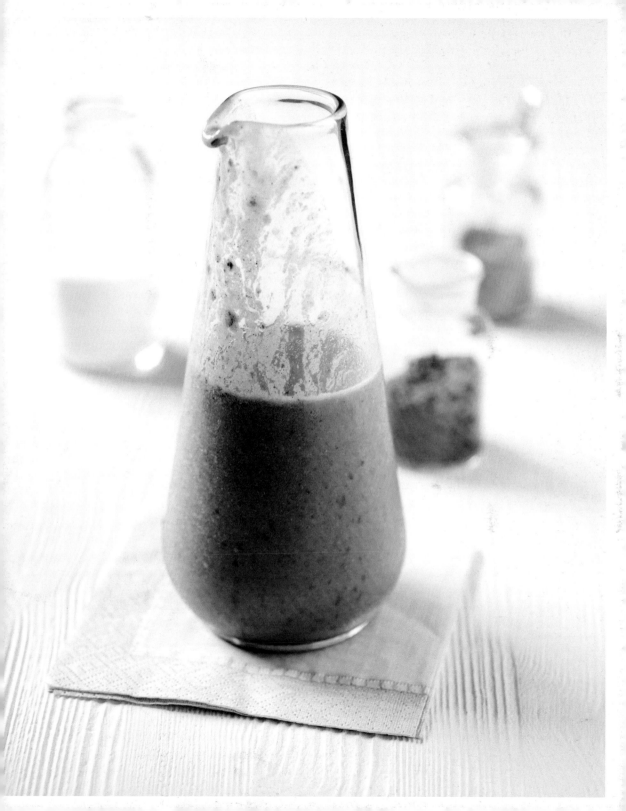

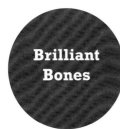

Brilliant Bones

Pictured>

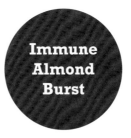

Immune Almond Burst

1 tbsp almonds
2 Brazil nuts
1 tbsp cashew nuts
1 tsp sesame seeds
½ tsp BAOBAB powder
1 tbsp COLLAGEN powder
2 dried, ready-to-eat figs
2 pitted soft dried dates
½ tsp ground cinnamon
1 tsp vanilla extract

Calcium- and magnesium-rich ingredients make this a first-class smoothie for healthy bones. Dried figs and dates contain calcium and soluble fibre. Baobab contains vitamin C, vital for the production of collagen and essential for bone and tissue health.

Put the nuts and seeds in a blender or food processor and add 200ml/7fl oz/ scant 1 cup water. Blend until smooth. Add the remaining ingredients and blend until smooth and creamy. Serve immediately.

   (G) (D) (S) (CI)

Nutritional information per serving
Kcals 416 | **Protein** 27g
Carbohydrates 76.5g, of which sugars 17.2g
Fat 21.1g, of which saturates 3.2g

100g/3½oz/½ cup frozen pitted cherries
1 handful of kale or spinach
1 tbsp almond butter
½ tsp WHEATGRASS powder
½ tsp CHAGA powder or MACA powder
1 tbsp DRIED MULBERRIES, or
    INCAN BERRIES or GOJI BERRIES
½ tsp ACAI BERRY powder
2 tsp vanilla extract
200ml/7fl oz/scant 1 cup COCONUT
    WATER or water

Superfruits, plus supergreens, are key ingredients in this immune-supporting blend. The cherries and almond butter combine to produce a smooth, comforting and creamy texture.

Put all the ingredients into a blender or food processor and blend until smooth and creamy. Serve immediately.

(G) (D) (S) (SE) (CI) (V)

Nutritional information per serving
Kcals 211 | **Protein** 5.6g
Carbohydrates 22.9g, of which sugars 12.6g
Fat 11.4g, of which saturates 0.9g

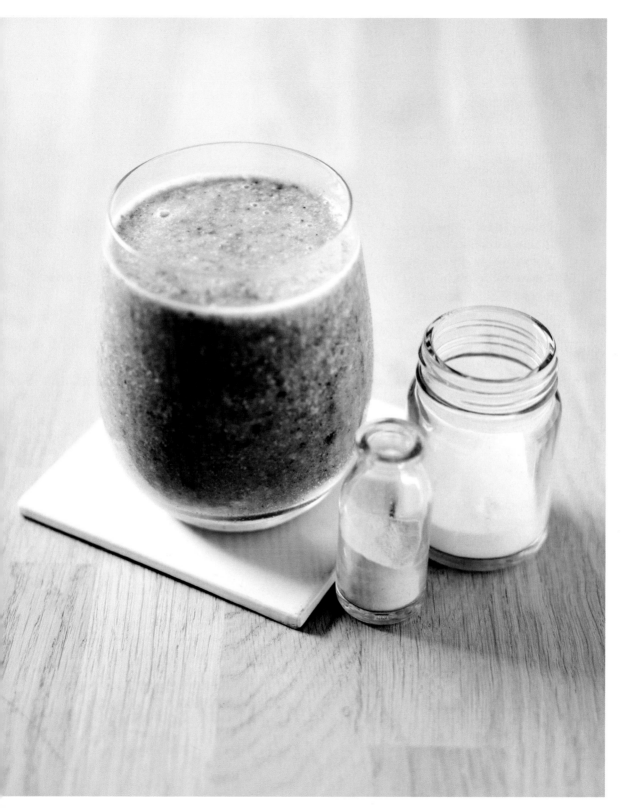

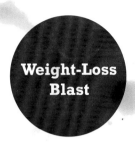

Weight-Loss Blast

125ml/4fl oz/½ cup brewed **GREEN COFFEE** powder, regular coffee or dandelion/
  chicory coffee
125ml/4fl oz/½ cup **COCONUT WATER or water**
1 tbsp cashew nuts
1 tsp ground cinnamon
2 tsp vanilla extract
a pinch of cayenne pepper
1 tsp **MACA** powder
1 tbsp **RAW CACAO** powder
½ tsp **CHIA SEEDS**
½ tsp **COCONUT OIL**, melted
a little stevia, if needed, to taste
4 ice cubes

As part of your weight-loss programme, take this smoothie containing green coffee
extract, which has been shown to enhance weight loss and boost the metabolism.
Another metabolism booster is coconut oil, but don't be concerned that adding fats
will make you fat; coconut oil has also been shown to stabilize blood sugar levels –
another essential way to control weight gain. This smoothie is sustaining because it
contains chia seeds to keep you feeling fuller for longer. Green coffee is available as
a powder, but you can make it up like regular coffee for this drink. If unavailable, use
regular coffee or green tea plus a spoonful of chicory or dandelion coffee for flavour.

Put all the ingredients, except the ice, into a blender or food processor and blend until
smooth and creamy. Add the ice and blend briefly to retain some texture. Serve immediately.

(G) (D) (S) (CI) (V)

Nutritional information per serving
Kcals 194 | **Protein** 6.8g
Carbohydrates 17.9g, of which sugars 0.7g
Fat 10.7g, of which saturates 3.4g

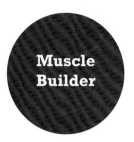

Muscle Builder

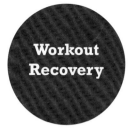

Workout Recovery

1 small banana
1 tbsp **RAW CACAO** powder
2 tbsp **CHOCOLATE PROTEIN** powder
1 tbsp crunchy natural peanut butter
1 tbsp **GLUTAMINE** powder
1 tsp **MACA** powder
1 tbsp **COLOSTRUM** powder (optional)
250ml/9fl oz/1 cup almond milk
4 ice cubes

½ banana
70g/2½oz/⅓ cup frozen pitted cherries
1 tbsp **COLOSTRUM** powder or **GLUTAMINE** powder
1 tsp **PROBIOTIC** powder
1 tbsp **PROTEIN** powder
250ml/9fl oz/1 cup **COCONUT WATER**
2 tbsp **CHOCOLATE PROTEIN** powder
4 ice cubes

This smoothie is high in protein and glutamine, and is designed to improve recovery after training. Peanuts contain mono-unsaturated fats, magnesium, potassium and vitamins E and B6.

Colostrum is the ultimate food to follow a workout. The natural compounds and growth factors in colostrum support the growth and repair of cells and tissues, resulting in faster recovery time after intense training.

Chop the banana and put it into a freezer bag. Exclude all the air, then seal and freeze overnight or until solid. Put the banana into a blender or food processor and add the remaining ingredients except the ice. Blend until smooth and creamy. Add the ice and blend briefly to retain some texture. Serve the smoothie immediately.

Chop the banana and put it into a freezer bag. Exclude all the air, then seal and freeze overnight or until solid. Put the banana into a blender or food processor and add the remaining ingredients except the ice. Blend until smooth and creamy. Add the ice and blend until smooth. Serve immediately.

  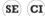

Nutritional information per serving
Kcals 478 | **Protein** 36.9g
Carbohydrates 55.5g, of which sugars 16.6g
Fat 16g, of which saturates 2.1g

Nutritional information per serving
Kcals 262 | **Protein** 22.5g
Carbohydrates 33.4g, of which sugars 15.6g
Fat 5g, of which saturates 0g

Longevity
Iced
Cream

30g/1oz/scant ¼ cup cashew nuts
1 tbsp **GOJI BERRIES**
2 tsp **MANUKA** or **RAW HONEY**
1 tsp **VANILLA PROTEIN** powder
1 tsp **PROBIOTIC** powder
3 tbsp **LUCUMA** powder
½ tsp **HE SHOU WU** powder, or **MEDICINAL MUSHROOM** powder or **MACA** powder
1 tsp **COCONUT OIL**, melted
1 tsp **MACA** powder
½ tsp ground cinnamon
1 tsp **LECITHIN** granules
8 ice cubes

This thick, iced smoothie is crammed with anti-ageing ingredients. He shou wu is an ancient Chinese longevity tonic, which helps to strengthen the organs, particularly the kidneys and liver. Available as a powder, either on its own or in vitality blends, he shou wu is an excellent rejuvenator for the whole body.

Put the nuts, goji berries and 125ml/4fl oz/½ cup water into a blender or food processor and blend until smooth. Add the remaining ingredients, except the ice, and blend until smooth and creamy. Add the ice and blend until thick – almost like soft ice cream. Serve immediately and eat with a spoon.

Health Benefits
Lecithin granules are a good source of choline, which helps the body to produce acetylcholine, a substance that acts as a chemical messenger to parts of the nervous system, and is essential to the brain's memory function. Choline is an essential fat in the body's cell membranes and helps to make up the protective sheaths surrounding the nerve cells.

Nutritional information per serving
Kcals 421 | **Protein** 8.4g
Carbohydrates 51.5g, of which sugars 22.4g
Fat 18.3g, of which saturates 5.4g

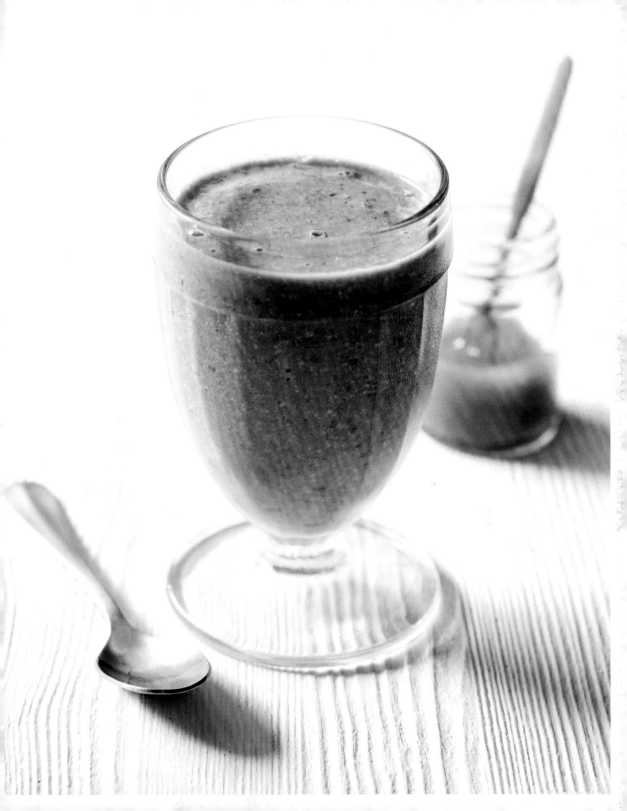

Strawberry Macadamia Shake

Pictured>

Rhubarb and Strawberry Shake

½ banana
1 tbsp macadamia nuts
5 strawberries, stalks discarded,
    chopped, or frozen mixed berries
1 tsp MIXED SUPERFOOD BERRY
    powder or ACAI BERRY powder

Try this quick and simple creamy
milkshake – perfect for the summer
when strawberries are in season. If fresh
strawberries are not available, however,
make use of mixed frozen berries or
raspberries instead. For an additional
supercharged shot, the shake includes
a spoonful of berry superfood powder.

Chop the banana and put it into a freezer
bag. Exclude all the air, then seal and freeze
overnight or until solid. Put the banana into
a blender or food processor and add the
remaining ingredients and 200ml/7fl oz/
scant 1 cup water. Blend until smooth and
creamy. Serve immediately.

      G D S SE CI V

Nutritional information per serving
Kcals 179 | **Protein** 2.1g
Carbohydrates 13.3g, of which sugars 12g
Fat 12.8g, of which saturates 1.7g

100g/3½oz/⅔ cup strawberries, stalks
    discarded, or frozen strawberries
60g/2¼oz rhubarb, fresh or frozen
1 tsp MANUKA or RAW HONEY
150ml/5fl oz/scant ⅔ cup tinned
    low-fat coconut milk, MILK KEFIR
    or COCONUT KEFIR (page 22)
100ml/3½fl oz/generous ⅓ cup
    POMEGRANATE juice

Slightly tart from the rhubarb, this
smoothie is rather like a rhubarb and
strawberry pie with just the right amount
of sweetness. If you prefer an extra-
creamy shake, use full-fat coconut milk
or dairy milk. Or for a high-probiotic
version, choose coconut kefir.

Put all the ingredients into a blender or
food processor and blend until smooth
and creamy. Serve immediately.

   G D S SE CI

Nutritional information per serving
Kcals 124 | **Protein** 1.9g
Carbohydrates 22.5g, of which sugars 22.5g
Fat 2.9g, of which saturates 0g

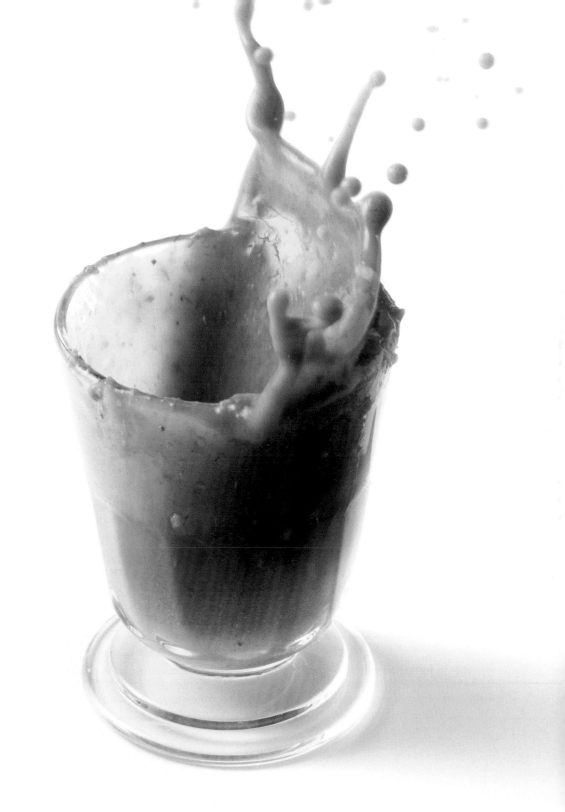

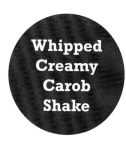

Whipped Creamy Carob Shake

1 banana
3 tbsp SHELLED HEMP SEEDS
½ tsp ground cinnamon
2 pitted soft dried dates
1 tbsp CAROB powder
1 tsp vanilla extract

FOR THE WHIPPED CREAMY TOPPING
400ml/14fl oz/1½ cups tinned full-fat
   coconut milk
2 tbsp xylitol
1 tsp vanilla extract
a little cinnamon, for dusting

This shake is topped with whipped coconut cream. Carob – technically a legume – is rich in fibre, B vitamins, vitamin E and antioxidants. Hemp seeds provide essential omega-3 fats to support brain function. The topping will keep for 3 days in the fridge.

Chop the banana and put it into a freezer bag. Exclude all the air, then seal and freeze overnight or until solid. Chill the tin of coconut milk for the topping upright in the fridge overnight. Put a glass bowl in the fridge so that it becomes very cold.

Grind the xylitol for the topping in a food processor or grinder until fine. Transfer to a small bowl and leave to one side. Put the hemp seeds into the food processor or blender and add 250ml/9fl oz/1 cup water. Blend until smooth. Add the banana and the remaining smoothie ingredients. Blend until smooth and creamy. Pour into a glass. To make the topping, open the tin of coconut milk and scoop off the top layer of solid coconut, then put it into the chilled bowl. Save the remaining coconut liquid for another recipe. Whisk the milk with a hand-held electric mixer on high speed for 15–20 seconds. Sift in the xylitol and stir in the vanilla. Scoop a spoonful over the top of the smoothie and dust with cinnamon. Serve immediately.

(G) (D) (S) (CI) (V)

Nutritional information per serving
Kcals 403 | **Protein** 17.3g
Carbohydrates 31.2g, of which sugars 26.4g
Fat 23.5g, of which saturates 5.8g

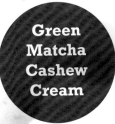

Green Matcha Cashew Cream

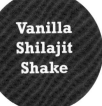

Vanilla Shilajit Shake

2 tbsp cashew nuts

3 pitted soft dried dates

1 handful of frozen or fresh raw, podded peas

1 handful of spinach leaves

1 tsp COCONUT OIL, melted

¼ tsp MATCHA GREEN TEA powder

½ tsp MACA powder

1 tsp CHIA SEEDS

150ml/5fl oz/scant ⅔ cup almond milk (page 21) or other dairy-free milk alternative

4 COCONUT ICE CUBES (page 22) or ice cubes

Cashew nuts make a perfect base for enriched non-dairy smoothies. Here, green vegetables and healthful powders make a nutritious iced drink.

Put all the ingredients, except the ice, into a blender or food processor and blend until smooth and creamy. Add the ice and blend briefly to retain some texture. Serve the smoothie immediately.

(G) (D) (S) (CI) (V)

Nutritional information per serving
Kcals 206 | **Protein** 6.6g
Carbohydrates 16.3g, of which sugars 5.1g
Fat 12.9g, of which saturates 4.2g

30g/1oz/scant ¼ cup cashew nuts

2 tsp MANUKA or RAW HONEY

2 tsp vanilla extract

1 tsp TOCOTRIENOLS or 1 vitamin E capsule, plus the squeezed capsule

2 tsp COCONUT OIL, melted

½ tsp SHILAJIT powder

1 tsp BEE POLLEN (optional)

250ml/9fl oz/1 cup COCONUT WATER or water

This silky vanilla and cashew-nut shake is sweetened with a little honey and bee pollen, both of which provide potent anti-microbial healing benefits. Shilajit powder contains over 88 dietary minerals and trace minerals – the full spectrum needed for human health. One of these is humic acid, a powerful anti-viral compound, which is beneficial for the immune system.

Put all the ingredients into a blender or food processor and blend until smooth and creamy. Serve immediately.

(G) (D) (S) (SE) (CI)

Nutritional information per serving
Kcals 306 | **Protein** 7.8g
Carbohydrates 21.3g, of which sugars 7.1g
Fat 21.1g, of which saturates 8.1g

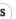

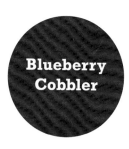

Blueberry Cobbler

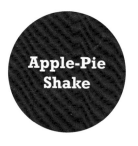

Apple-Pie Shake

6 pecan nut halves, finely chopped
2 tbsp porridge oats
60g/2¼oz/heaped ⅓ cup fresh or frozen
    blueberries
½ apple, cored and chopped
60ml/2fl oz/¼ cup apple juice
½ tsp ground cinnamon
½ tsp COCONUT OIL
60g/2¼oz/¼ cup natural yogurt or soya
    yogurt
100ml/3½fl oz/generous ⅓ cup dairy
    or COCONUT KEFIR (page 22), semi-
    skimmed milk or milk alternative

To make the cobbler mix, put the nuts and
oats in a dry frying pan over a medium
heat and toast until lightly golden, stirring
frequently. Leave to cool. Put all the
remaining ingredients into a blender or
food processor and blend until smooth
and creamy. Add most of the cobbler mix
and blend again until smooth. Stir in the
remaining cobbler mix, then serve. Eat
with a spoon.

Nutritional information per serving
Kcals 338 | **Protein** 8.5g
Carbohydrates 36.8g, of which sugars 18.4g
Fat 17.4g, of which saturates 2.7g

200ml/7fl oz/scant 1 cup cashew milk
    or almond milk (page 21)
3 walnut halves
1 small apple, cored and chopped
½ tsp vanilla extract
2 pitted soft dried dates
½ tsp ground cinnamon
½ tsp MACA powder
a pinch of freshly grated nutmeg or
    cinnamon, for dusting
a pinch of ground allspice, for dusting

**Apples are a great source of pectin – a
soluble fibre shown to benefit digestive
health. Cinnamon is an excellent spice
for balancing blood sugar levels, and
walnuts contain protein and healthy
essential omega-3 fats.**

Put all the ingredients into a blender or
food processor and blend until smooth
and creamy. Pour into a glass and dust
over a little nutmeg and allspice. Serve
the smoothie immediately.

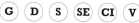

Nutritional information per serving
Kcals 210 | **Protein** 3.5g
Carbohydrates 20.9g, of which sugars 11.8g
Fat 12.4g, of which saturates 1.1g

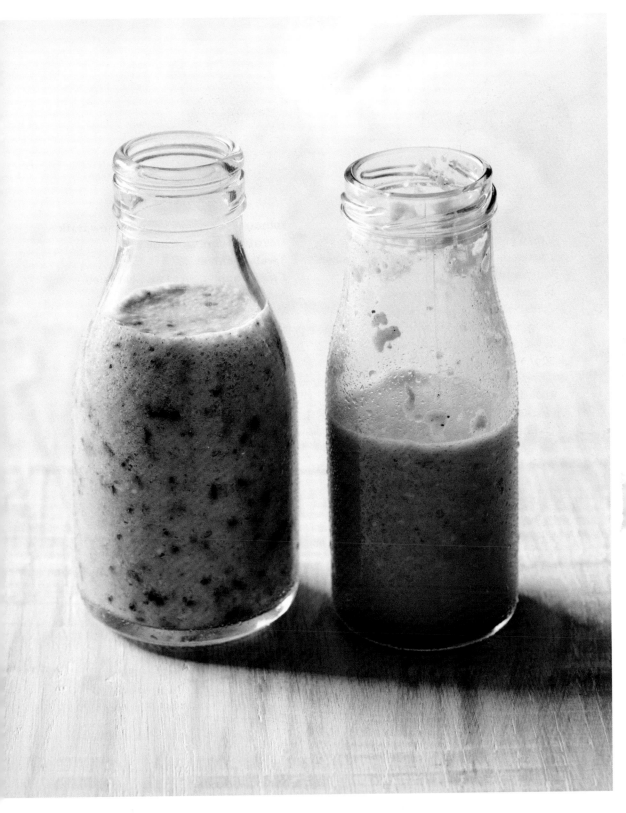

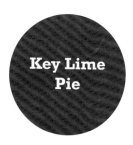

Key Lime Pie

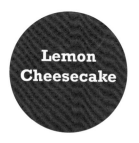

Lemon Cheesecake

1 small banana
1 tbsp avocado
1 lime, peeled and deseeded
½ tsp vanilla extract
½ tsp WHEATGRASS powder or
   BARLEY GRASS powder
1 tsp MANUKA or RAW HONEY, or to taste
200ml/7fl oz/scant 1 cup almond milk
   (page 21)

With a dash of sharpness, just like a key lime pie, and with the richness of almond milk, this smoothie is high in health-giving foods. A thick texture is achieved by blending frozen banana with a spoonful of avocado for added enrichment. For an indulgent addition, pour in 1 teaspoon melted cacao butter.

Chop the banana and put it into a freezer bag. Exclude all the air, then seal and freeze overnight or until solid. Put the banana into a blender or food processor and add the remaining ingredients. Blend until smooth and creamy. Serve immediately.

G **D** **S** **SE**

Nutritional information per serving
Kcals 178 | **Protein** 2.1g
Carbohydrates 29.5g, of which sugars 19.1g
Fat 5.2g, of which saturates 0.7g

½ banana
150ml/5fl oz/scant ⅔ cup
   COCONUT WATER
3 pitted soft dried dates
2 tbsp cashew nuts
1 lemon, peeled and deseeded
zest of 1 lemon
2 tbsp VANILLA PROTEIN powder
2 tsp LUCUMA powder
½ tsp vanilla extract
4 ice cubes

An icy-cold lemon cheesecake in a glass, this smoothie is high in protein and makes a tasty and energizing drink – ideal as a post-workout snack.

Chop the banana and put it into a freezer bag. Exclude all the air, then seal and freeze overnight or until solid. Put the banana into a blender or food processor and add the remaining ingredients except the ice. Blend until smooth and creamy. Add the ice and blend until smooth and creamy. Serve the smoothie immediately.

G **S** **SE**

Nutritional information per serving
Kcals 315 | **Protein** 19.6g
Carbohydrates 33.2g, of which sugars 16.5g
Fat 11.2g, of which saturates 1.2g

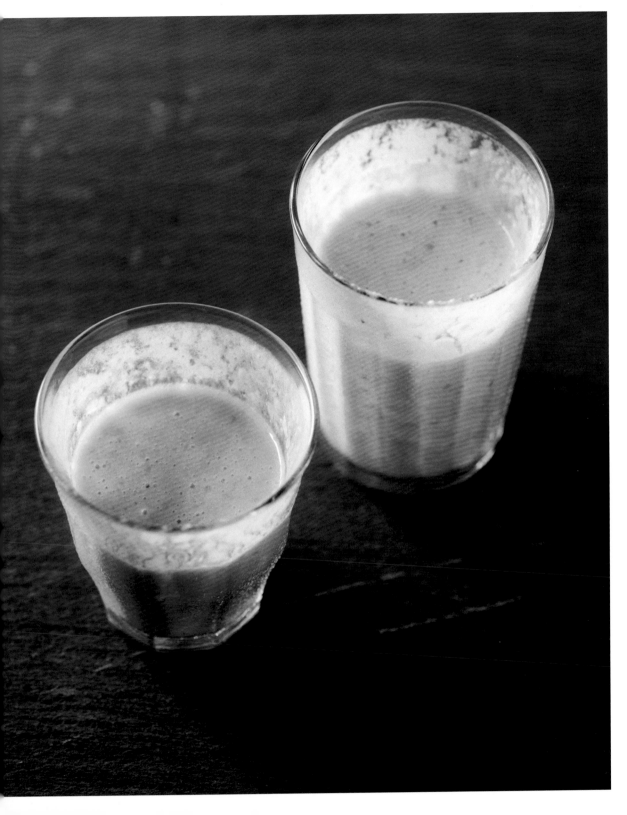

Lime Kefir Cream

100ml/3½fl oz/generous ⅓ cup **MILK KEFIR** or **COCONUT KEFIR** (page 22)
100ml/3½fl oz/generous ⅓ cup full-fat coconut milk
1 tbsp mint leaves, chopped
1 tsp **MANUKA** or **RAW HONEY**
1 tsp **BEE POLLEN**, or **RAW** or **MANUKA HONEY**
zest of 1 lime
1 tsp **WHEATGRASS** powder or **SPIRULINA** powder
1 lime, peeled, deseeded and chopped
4 ice cubes or **COCONUT ICE CUBES** (page 22)

The kefir and lime combine to give this luscious shake a delicious tangy and tart flavour. Any green superfood would work well in this smoothie, but for a higher protein content try a little spirulina powder.

Put all the ingredients, except the ice, into a blender or food processor and blend until smooth and creamy. Add the ice and blend briefly to retain some texture. Serve immediately.

Nutritional information per serving
Kcals 105 | **Protein** 6.4g
Carbohydrates 15.3g, of which sugars 7.7g
Fat 1.3g, of which saturates 0.3g

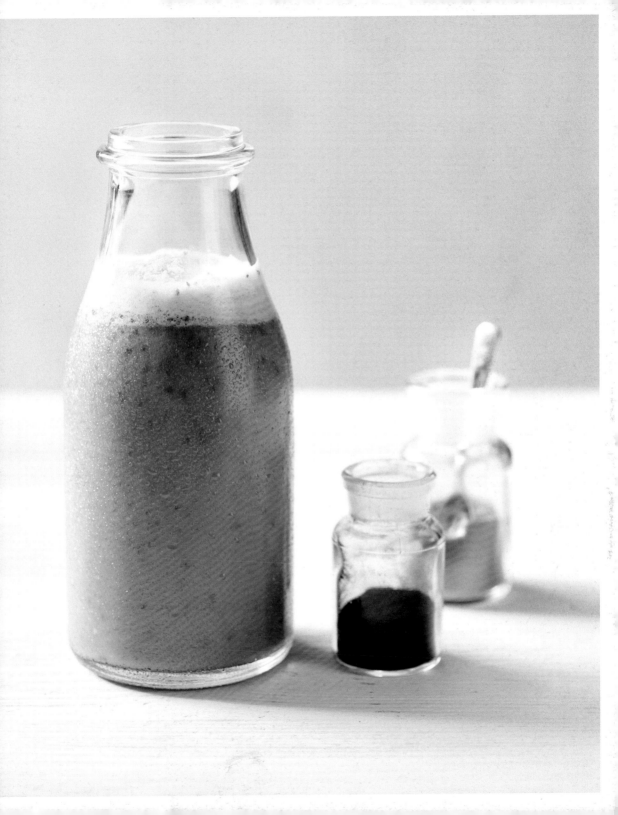

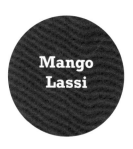

Mango
Lassi

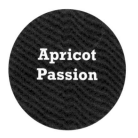

Apricot
Passion

½ mango, peeled and chopped
150ml/5fl oz/scant ⅔ cup
    COCONUT WATER
1 tsp COCONUT OIL, melted
2 tbsp desiccated coconut
1 tsp lemon juice
a pinch of Himalayan sea salt or sea salt
a pinch of ground cardamom, for dusting
    (optional)

Refreshing and fruity, this Indian drink is
perfect to serve as a dessert. A spoonful
of coconut oil provides healthy medium-
chain triglycerides, which are readily
burnt by the body, making this an ideal
drink for energy.

Put all the ingredients, except the
cardamom, if using, into a blender or
food processor and blend until smooth
and creamy. Dust with a little cardamom,
if you like, and serve immediately.

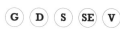

Nutritional information per serving
Kcals 174 | **Protein** 2.3g
Carbohydrates 16.8g, of which sugars 11.3g
Fat 10.9g, of which saturates 9.1g

50g/1¾oz silken tofu, mashed
2 ready-to-eat dried apricots, chopped
100ml/3½fl oz/generous ⅓ cup freshly
    squeezed orange juice
1 tsp orange zest
100ml/3½fl oz/generous ⅓ cup
    COCONUT WATER
¼ tsp BAOBAB powder
2 fresh apricots, pitted and chopped

For a great source of protein, mix up this
silky, dairy-free smoothie containing
silken tofu. Dried apricots increase
the soluble fibre and give the drink
a wonderful sweetness.

Put all the ingredients into a blender or
food processor and blend until smooth
and creamy. Serve immediately.

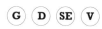

Nutritional information per serving
Kcals 132 | **Protein** 6.4g
Carbohydrates 21g, of which sugars 17.5g
Fat 2.5g, of which saturates 0.3g

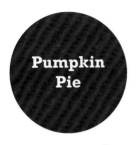

Pumpkin Pie

½ banana
100g/3½oz/⅓ cup tinned pumpkin purée, or cooked pumpkin, puréed
½ tsp ground cinnamon
200ml/7fl oz/scant 1 cup almond milk (page 21)
1 tbsp SHELLED HEMP SEEDS
1 tsp vanilla extract
2 tbsp VANILLA HEMP or PEA PROTEIN powder
4 ice cubes
coconut sugar (optional), to taste

Puréed pumpkin works exceptionally well in smoothies, because it has a slightly sweet flavour and its texture adds body to the drink. Combined with hemp seeds and almond milk, it's full of nourishment and has tasty, warm overtones from the cinnamon. Adding protein powder provides additional protein and helps to stabilize blood sugar levels.

Chop the banana and put it into a freezer bag. Exclude all the air, then seal and freeze overnight or until solid. Put the banana into a blender or food processor and add the remaining ingredients except the ice and sugar. Blend until smooth and creamy. Add the ice and blend briefly to retain some texture. Sweeten to taste, if needed. Serve immediately.

(G) (D) (S) (CI) (V)

Nutritional information per serving
Kcals 279 | **Protein** 20.4g
Carbohydrates 23.8g, of which sugars 9.7g
Fat 11.3g, of which saturates 0.5g

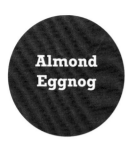

Almond Eggnog

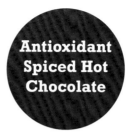

Antioxidant Spiced Hot Chocolate

250ml/9fl oz/1 cup almond milk or
    cashew milk (page 21)
1 tbsp macadamia nuts
1 small banana, peeled and chopped
2 pitted soft dried dates
½ tsp BEE POLLEN, or RAW or
    MANUKA HONEY
1 tsp vanilla extract
a pinch of freshly grated nutmeg
¼ tsp ground cinnamon, plus extra
    for dusting
a pinch of ground cloves

Deliciously creamy eggnog is a seasonal
favourite. The use of nut milk and
macadamia nuts in this version adds
protein, magnesium and calcium for
bone health. For an extra vitamin C boost,
add ½ teaspoon baobab powder.

Put all the ingredients into a blender or
food processor and blend until smooth and
creamy. Serve immediately, dusted with a
little ground cinnamon.

Nutritional information per serving
Kcals 276 | **Protein** 3.4g
Carbohydrates 32.6g, of which sugars 20.4g
Fat 14.6g, of which saturates 1.9g

200ml/7fl oz/scant 1 cup full-fat
    coconut milk
a large pinch of ground TURMERIC
a pinch of chilli powder or cayenne
    pepper
1 cinnamon stick
1 cardamom pod, crushed
1 thin slice of root ginger, peeled
2 tsp coconut sugar, or to taste
a pinch of Himalayan sea salt or sea salt
2 tsp RAW CACAO powder
½ tsp MACA powder
½ tsp vanilla extract
1 PROPOLIS capsule, contents tipped
    in and capsule added (optional)

Put the coconut milk in a saucepan over
a medium heat and add 3 tablespoons hot
water. Add the turmeric, chilli powder,
cinnamon, cardamom, ginger, sugar and salt,
and bring gently to the boil. Reduce the heat
and simmer, very gently, for 5 minutes. Strain
the milk into a blender or food processor.
Add the remaining ingredients, then blend
until smooth and creamy. Serve.

Nutritional information per serving
Kcals 106 | **Protein** 2.8g
Carbohydrates 22.7g, of which sugars 15g
Fat 1.6g, of which saturates 1g

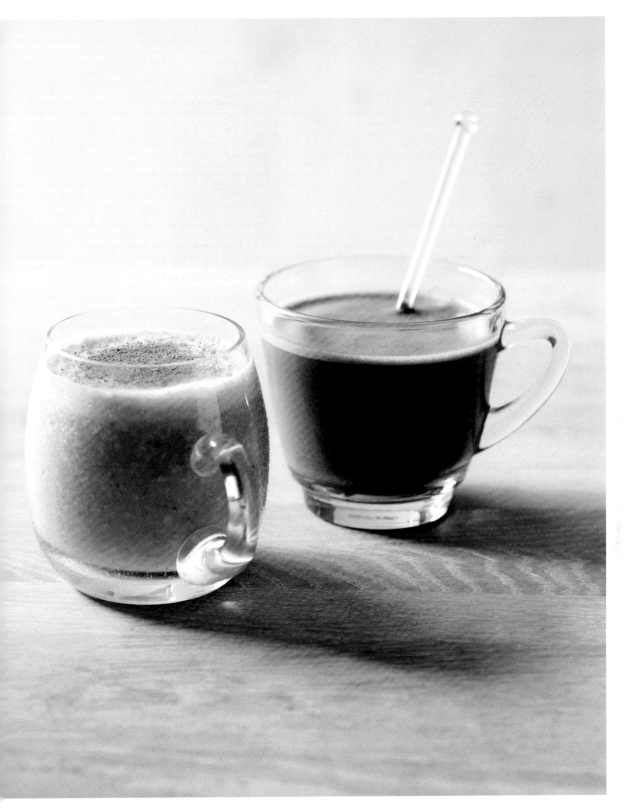

The Quick Look

W **Weight loss (fat-burner)** The drinks are graded as: 5 stars (200 calories or less) – best for weight loss; 4 stars (201–250 calories); 3 stars (251–300 calories).

C **Cleansing (encompassing detoxing and digestion)** To help support the detoxification system and the removal of toxins. They are also soothing for the digestive system.

R **Radiance (anti-ageing)** Containing known 'beauty nutrients' to promote youthful, glowing skin, nails and hair as well as possessing anti-ageing properties.

E **Energy** To boost performance and energy levels, for balancing blood sugar and with nutrients for sustained energy and to enhance muscle mass.

I **Immune boost** To support the body's immune system. The drinks contain ingredients that have anti-microbial and anti-viral properties.

B **Brain health and stress** For brain and cognitive health, including vitamins, minerals, healthy fats and antioxidants essential for optimal brain function.

Juices

Grapefruit Greens (page 26)

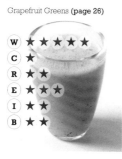

W ★★★★★
C ★
R ★★
E ★★★
I ★★
B ★★

Morning Blend (page 26)

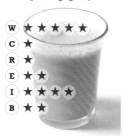

W ★★★★★
C ★
R ★
E ★★
I ★★★★
B ★★

Creamy C Revitalizer (page 28)

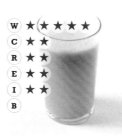

W ★★★★★
C ★★
R ★★
E ★★
I ★★
B

Blue Guava (page 30)

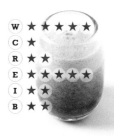

W ★★★★★
C ★
R ★★
E ★★★★
I ★★
B ★★

Tropics Blend (page 30)

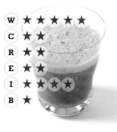

W ★★★★★
C ★★
R ★★
E ★★
I ★★★
B ★

Spicy Golden Lemonade (page 32)

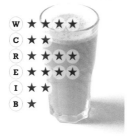

W ★★★★
C ★★
R ★★★
E ★★★
I ★★
B ★

Cranberry Burst (page 33)

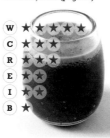

W ★★★★★
C ★★★
R ★★★
E
I ★
B ★

Orange and Peach Buckthorn Crush (page 33)

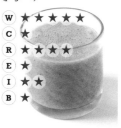

W ★★★★
C ★
R ★★★
E ★
I ★★
B ★

Plum and Orange Spice **(page 34)**
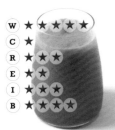
W ★★★★★
C ★
R ★★★
E ★★
I ★★★
B ★★★

Hot Spiced Apple **(page 34)**
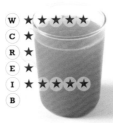
W ★★★★★
C ★
R ★
E ★
I ★★★★★
B

Apple-Cinnamon Aid **(page 36)**
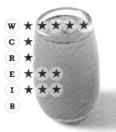
W ★★★★★
C ★
R ★
E ★★
I ★★
B

Gingered Melon **(page 36)**
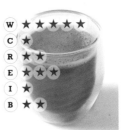
W ★★★★★
C ★
R ★★
E ★★
I ★
B ★★

Apricot Immune **(page 38)**
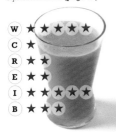
W ★★★★★
C ★
R ★★
E ★★
I ★★★
B ★★★

Red Sour **(page 40)**
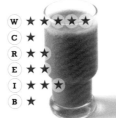
W ★★★★★
C ★
R ★★
E ★
I ★★
B ★

Berry Kombucha **(page 41)**
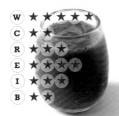
W ★★★★★
C ★★
R ★★★
E ★★★★
I ★★★
B ★★

Strawberry Fizz **(page 42)**
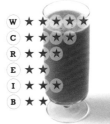
W ★★★★★
C ★★★
R ★★★
E
I ★★★
B ★★

Summer Berry Peach **(page 42)**
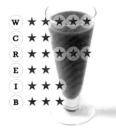
W ★★★★★
C ★★
R ★★★★★
E ★★
I ★★★
B ★★★

Acai Berry Refresher **(page 44)**
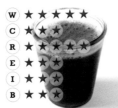
W ★★★★★
C ★★★
R ★★★★★
E ★★★
I ★★★
B ★★★

Sweet Greens **(page 46)**
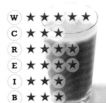
W ★★★★★
C ★★
R ★★★★
E ★★★★
I ★★★
B ★★★

Berry Greens **(page 46)**
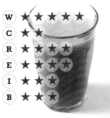
W ★★★★★
C ★★
R ★★★★
E ★★★★
I ★★★
B ★★★

Skin Protector **(page 48)**
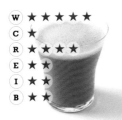
W ★★★★★
C ★
R ★★★
E ★★
I ★★
B ★★

Digestive Aid **(page 49)**
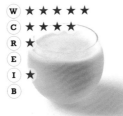
W ★★★★★
C ★★★★
R ★
E
I
B

Cellulite Cleanse **(page 49)**
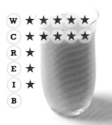
W ★★★★★
C ★★★★★
R ★
E ★
I ★
B ★

Natural Anti-Inflammatory Fighter **(page 50)**
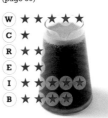
W ★★★★★
C ★
R ★★
E ★★
I ★★★★★
B ★★★★

Chlorophyll Wonder (**page 54**)

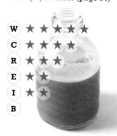

Electrolyte Burst (**page 54**)

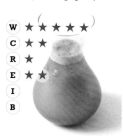

Veggie Cleansing Combo (**page 56**)

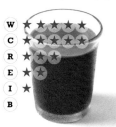

Romaine Lemon Twister (**page 56**)

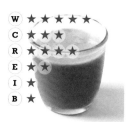

Lemon Green Cleanser (**page 58**)

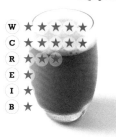

Broccoli Pear Crush (**page 60**)

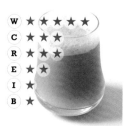

Spinach Blend (**page 61**)

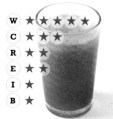

Sweet Kale (**page 61**)

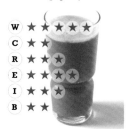

Ginger Green Combo (**page 62**)

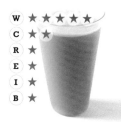

Salad Shake (**page 62**)

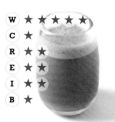

Digestion Comforter (**page 64**)

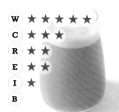

Stomach Soother (**page 64**)

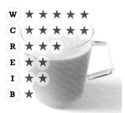

Inflammatory Aid (**page 66**)

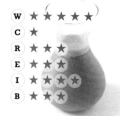

Root Lift (**page 68**)

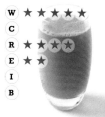

Skin Clear (**page 68**)

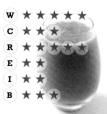

Pepper Burst (**page 70**)

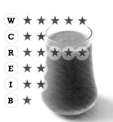

Red Beauty **(page 70)**

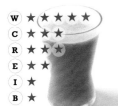

W ★ ★ ★ ★ ★
C ★ ★ ★
R ★ ★ ★ ★
E ★ ★
I ★
B ★

Cellulite Buster **(page 71)**

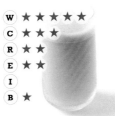

W ★ ★ ★ ★ ★
C ★ ★ ★
R ★ ★
E ★ ★
I ★
B ★

Iron Fortifier **(page 72)**

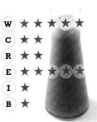

W ★ ★ ★ ★ ★
C ★ ★
R ★ ★
E ★ ★ ★ ★ ★
I ★
B ★

Fertility Boost **(page 74)**

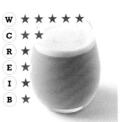

W ★ ★ ★ ★ ★
C ★ ★
R ★
E ★
I ★
B ★

Stamina Shot **(page 75)**

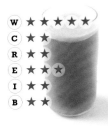

W ★ ★ ★ ★ ★
C ★ ★
R ★ ★
E ★ ★ ★
I ★ ★
B ★ ★

Rejuvenating Aloe Juice **(page 75)**

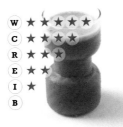

W ★ ★ ★ ★ ★
C ★ ★ ★ ★
R ★ ★ ★ ★
E ★ ★ ★
I ★
B

Sweet Beet Hydrator **(page 76)**

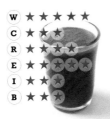

W ★ ★ ★ ★ ★
C ★ ★ ★
R ★ ★ ★ ★ ★
E ★ ★ ★ ★ ★
I ★ ★ ★ ★
B ★ ★ ★

Pumpkin Power **(page 76)**

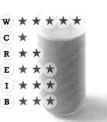

W ★ ★ ★ ★ ★
C ★
R ★ ★
E ★ ★ ★
I ★ ★ ★
B ★ ★ ★

Beet and Berry Performance
(page 78)

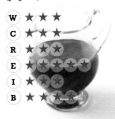

W ★ ★ ★
C ★ ★ ★
R ★ ★ ★
E ★ ★ ★ ★ ★
I ★ ★ ★
B ★ ★ ★

Coriander Detox **(page 80)**

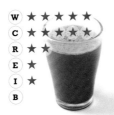

W ★ ★ ★ ★ ★
C ★ ★ ★ ★ ★
R ★ ★
E ★
I ★
B

Golden Blend **(page 80)**

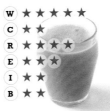

W ★ ★ ★ ★ ★
C ★ ★
R ★ ★ ★ ★
E ★ ★ ★
I ★ ★
B ★ ★

Smoothies

Avocado Greens **(page 84)**

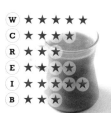

W ★★★★★
C ★★★★★
R ★★★
E ★★★★
I ★★★★★
B ★★★

Purple Greens **(page 84)**

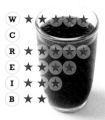

W ★★★★★
C ★
R ★★★★★
E ★★★★
I ★★★★★
B ★★

Brain Booster **(page 86)**

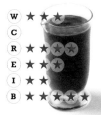

W ★★★
C ★
R ★★★★
E ★★★
I ★★
B ★★★★★

Minted Pea Greens **(page 88)**

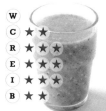

W ★
C ★★
R ★★★
E ★★★★★
I ★★★
B ★★

Green Machine **(page 89)**

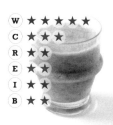

W ★★★★★
C ★★★
R ★★
E ★★
I ★★
B ★★

Spirulina Cream **(page 89)**

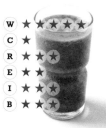

W ★★★★★
C ★
R ★★★
E ★★
I ★★
B ★★

Heavy Metal Detox **(page 90)**

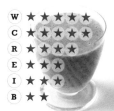

W ★★★★★
C ★★★★★
R ★★★
E ★★★
I ★★
B ★★

Savoury Blend **(page 90)**

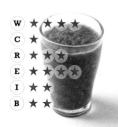

W ★★★
C ★★
R ★★
E ★★★
I ★★
B ★★

Joint Aid **(page 92)**

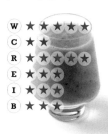

W ★★★★★
C ★★
R ★★★★★
E ★★★★
I ★★★
B ★★★

Gingered Pear Protein Support
(page 93)

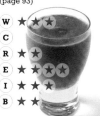

W ★★★
C ★
R ★★
E ★★★★★
I ★★★
B ★★

Magnesium Lift **(page 94)**

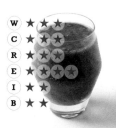

W ★★★
C ★★★
R ★★★★
E ★★★★
I ★★
B ★★

Matcha Green Tropical Blend
(page 96)

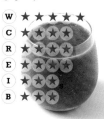

W ★★★★★
C ★★★★★
R ★★★★★
E ★★★★★
I ★★★★★
B ★★★

Pineapple Gazpacho **(page 96)**

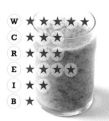

W ★★★★★
C ★★★
R ★★★
E ★★★★
I ★★★
B ★

Blackberry Rooibos **(page 97)**

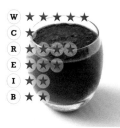

W ★★★★★
C ★
R ★★★★★
E ★★★★★
I ★★
B ★★

Iced Tea Protein Shake **(page 98)**

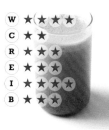

W ★★★★
C ★★
R ★
E ★★★
I ★★★
B ★★

Kombucha Smoother **(page 98)**

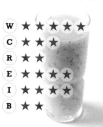

W ★★★★★
C ★★★
R ★★
E ★★★
I ★★★
B ★★

Chocolate Cinnamon Omega Elixir (page 100)

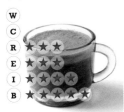

W
C
R ★ ★ ★
E ★ ★ ★
I ★ ★ ★
B ★ ★ ★

Carrot Spice (page 100)

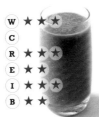

W ★ ★ ★
C
R ★ ★ ★
E ★ ★
I ★ ★ ★
B ★ ★

Chocolate Berry (page 102)

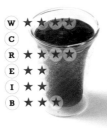

W ★ ★ ★ ★
C
R ★ ★ ★ ★
E ★ ★
I ★ ★
B ★ ★ ★

Beetroot Cake Crush (page 104)

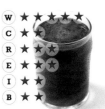

W ★ ★ ★ ★
C ★ ★
R ★ ★ ★
E ★ ★
I ★ ★
B ★ ★

Hormonal Energizer (page 105)

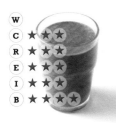

W
C ★ ★ ★
R ★ ★ ★
E ★ ★ ★
I ★ ★ ★
B ★ ★ ★

Goji Strawberry Smoothie (page 105)

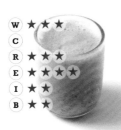

W ★ ★ ★
C
R ★ ★ ★
E ★ ★ ★ ★
I ★ ★
B ★ ★

Tropical Combo (page 106)

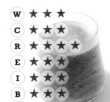

W ★ ★ ★
C ★ ★ ★
R ★ ★ ★
E ★ ★
I ★ ★ ★
B ★ ★ ★

Summer Tonic (page 106)

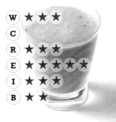

W ★ ★ ★
C
R ★ ★ ★
E ★ ★ ★ ★
I ★ ★ ★
B ★ ★

Super Fruits (page 108)

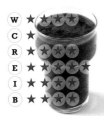

W ★ ★ ★ ★
C ★
R ★ ★ ★
E ★ ★ ★ ★
I ★ ★ ★
B ★ ★ ★

Orange Persimmon Blend (page 110)

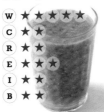

W ★ ★ ★ ★ ★
C ★ ★
R ★ ★
E ★ ★ ★
I ★ ★
B ★ ★

Green Dragon (page 110)

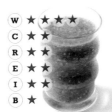

W ★ ★ ★ ★
C ★ ★
R ★ ★
E ★ ★
I ★ ★
B ★

Watermelon Crush (page 111)

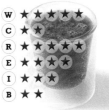

W ★ ★ ★ ★ ★
C ★ ★
R ★ ★ ★ ★ ★
E ★ ★ ★ ★
I ★ ★ ★
B ★ ★

Kefir Lime Colada (page 112)

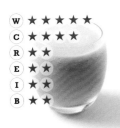

W ★ ★ ★ ★ ★
C ★ ★ ★ ★
R ★ ★
E ★ ★
I ★ ★
B ★ ★

Peachy Chia (page 112)

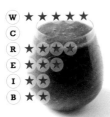

W ★ ★ ★ ★ ★
C
R ★ ★ ★ ★
E ★ ★ ★ ★
I
B ★ ★

Chocolate Hazelnut Cauliflower Cream (page 114)

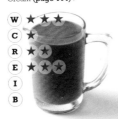

W ★ ★ ★
C ★
R ★ ★
E ★ ★ ★
I
B

Banana Pecan Stress Pick-Me-Up (page 114)

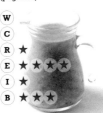

W
C
R ★
E ★ ★ ★ ★
I ★
B ★ ★ ★

Wake-Up Berry Latte **(page 118)**

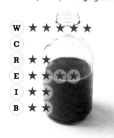

Kick-Start **(page 118)**

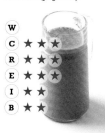

Creamy Superfood Mocha **(page 120)**

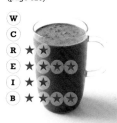

Breakfast Bowl **(page 122)**

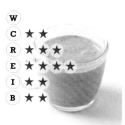

Espresso Shake **(page 123)**

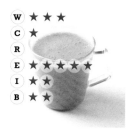

Banana Caramel Cream **(page 123)**

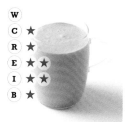

Chocolate Longevity Shake **(page 124)**

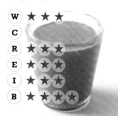

Shamrock Shake **(page 124)**

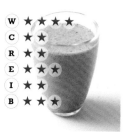

Ginger Stomach Soother **(page 126)**

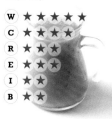

Liquorice Stress-Relief Smoothie **(page 126)**

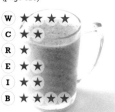

Joint-Health Greens **(page 128)**

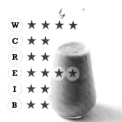

Brilliant Bones **(page 130)**

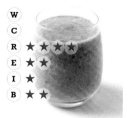

Immune Almond Burst **(page 130)**

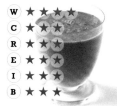

Weight-Loss Blast **(page 132)**

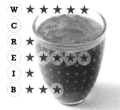

Muscle Builder **(page 133)**

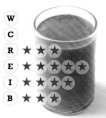

Workout Recovery **(page 133)**

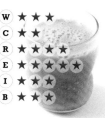

Longevity Iced Cream (page 134)

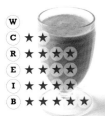

W
C ★ ★
R ★ ★ ★ ★
E ★ ★ ★ ★
I ★ ★ ★ ★
B ★ ★ ★ ★ ★

Strawberry Macadamia Shake (page 136)

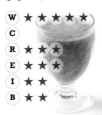

W ★ ★ ★ ★ ★
C
R ★ ★ ★
E ★ ★ ★
I ★ ★
B ★ ★

Rhubarb and Strawberry Shake (page 136)

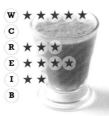

W ★ ★ ★ ★ ★
C
R ★ ★ ★
E ★ ★ ★ ★
I ★ ★
B ★

Whipped Creamy Carob Shake (page 138)

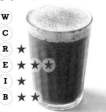

W
C
R ★
E ★ ★ ★
I ★
B ★ ★

Green Matcha Cashew Cream (page 139)

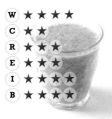

W ★ ★ ★ ★
C ★ ★
R ★ ★ ★
E ★ ★ ★
I ★ ★ ★ ★
B ★ ★ ★ ★

Vanilla Shilajit Shake (page 139)

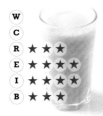

W
C
R ★ ★ ★
E ★ ★ ★ ★
I ★ ★ ★ ★
B ★ ★ ★

Blueberry Cobbler (page 140)

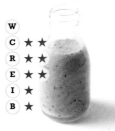

W
C ★ ★
R ★ ★
E ★ ★
I ★
B ★

Apple-Pie Shake (page 140)

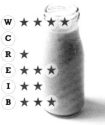

W ★ ★ ★ ★
C
R ★
E ★ ★ ★
I ★ ★
B ★ ★ ★

Key Lime Pie (page 142)

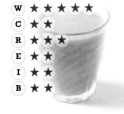

W ★ ★ ★ ★ ★
C ★ ★
R ★ ★ ★
E ★ ★
I ★ ★
B ★ ★

Lemon Cheesecake (page 142)

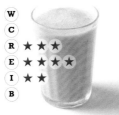

W
C
R ★ ★ ★
E ★ ★ ★ ★
I ★ ★
B

Lime Kefir Cream (page 144)

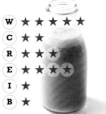

W ★ ★ ★ ★ ★
C ★ ★
R ★ ★ ★
E ★ ★ ★ ★
I ★
B ★

Mango Lassi (page 146)

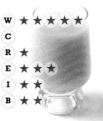

W ★ ★ ★ ★ ★
C
R ★
E ★ ★ ★
I ★ ★
B ★ ★

Apricot Passion (page 146)

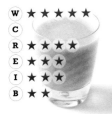

W ★ ★ ★ ★ ★
C
R ★ ★ ★ ★
E ★ ★ ★ ★
I ★ ★ ★
B ★ ★

Pumpkin Pie (page 147)

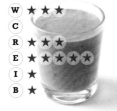

W ★ ★ ★
C
R ★ ★ ★
E ★ ★ ★ ★ ★
I ★
B ★

Almond Eggnog (page 148)

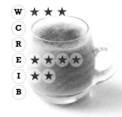

W ★ ★ ★
C
R
E ★ ★ ★ ★
I ★
B

Antioxidant Spiced Hot Chocolate (page 148)

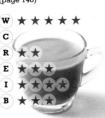

W ★ ★ ★ ★ ★
C
R ★ ★
E ★ ★ ★ ★
I ★ ★ ★ ★
B ★ ★ ★

Index

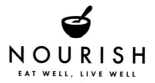

NOURISH
EAT WELL, LIVE WELL

Here at Nourish we're all about wellbeing through food and drink – irresistible dishes with a serious good-for-you factor. If you want to eat and drink delicious things that set you up for the day, suit any special diets, keep you healthy and make the most of the ingredients you have, we've got some great ideas to share with you. Come over to our blog for wholesome recipes and fresh inspiration – nourishbooks.com